AWAKEN YOUR BODY AWAKEN YOUR DESIRE

USING SCIENCE TO HEAL YOUR STRESS
& FIND YOUR SEXUAL VITALITY

DANIELLE ARMOUR, Ph.D.

Awaken Your Body, Awaken Your Desire
Using Science to Heal Your Stress & Find Your Sexual Vitality
By Danielle Armour, Ph.D.

Book cover by Kostis Pavlou
Artwork by Alan Syah

Copyright © 2025 by Danielle Armour. All rights reserved.

ISBN 979-8-9988651-0-7 (pbk.)
ISBN 979-8-9988651-1-4 (epub)
ISBN 979-8-9988651-2-1 (pdf)

Published by Eros & Evidence Publishing, LLC
Williamsburg, Virginia, 23188, U.S.A.
https://erosandevidence.com

DISCLAIMER

This book is intended for educational and informational purposes only. It is not intended to diagnose, treat, cure, or prevent any medical or psychological condition, nor is it a substitute for professional medical advice, diagnosis, or treatment.

The practices, exercises, and strategies described herein are based on the author's professional experience, training, and research in the fields of holistic healing and sexual wellness. While many readers may experience positive outcomes from these approaches, results are personal and may vary.

Always seek the advice of your physician, therapist, or qualified health provider with any questions you may have regarding a medical or mental health condition. Do not disregard professional medical advice or delay seeking it because of something you have read in this book.

The author and publisher disclaim all liability for any direct, indirect, incidental, or consequential loss or damage incurred by any reader as a result of the use or misuse of the information provided.

If you are in crisis or experiencing trauma-related distress, please seek immediate support from a licensed mental health professional or contact your local crisis center.

AWAKEN YOUR BODY AWAKEN YOUR DESIRE

DANIELLE ARMOUR, Ph.D.

Foreword by Laurie Mintz, Ph.D.

For over three decades, I've worked as a psychologist, professor, and sex therapist committed to helping women embrace their sexual pleasure without shame. Again and again, I've seen how misinformation, cultural conditioning, and everyday stress disconnect us from our bodies—and from the desire and satisfaction that are rightfully ours. The good news? There is a science to sexual well-being. And when we pair that science with self-compassion and embodiment, powerful things happen.

That's why I'm honored to introduce *Awaken Your Body, Awaken Your Desire*—a refreshingly wise and deeply grounded guide to reclaiming your sensual self. Danielle Armour brings together the best of research and lived insight to walk readers through the journey of returning to their bodies—not with judgment or pressure, but with kindness, curiosity, and clarity.

This is not another "how-to" book filled with performance-based advice. Instead, Danielle invites us to slow down, to listen inward, and to rediscover pleasure as something innate—not something earned or reserved for the perfect moment. Her tools—rooted in neuroscience, mindfulness, breathwork, and movement—are accessible, practical, and most importantly, human. They help us shift from sexual autopilot to awakened presence.

What makes this book stand out is its tone. It's smart, inclusive, and refreshingly shame-free. Danielle reminds us that pleasure isn't a luxury—it's a vital part of our overall health and happiness. Whether you've struggled with low desire, felt overwhelmed by stress, or simply want to reconnect with your sensual vitality, this book meets you where you are—and helps you move forward with confidence.

If you've ever wondered where your desire went—or whether it's even possible to get it back—Danielle has answers. More than that, she offers a path to remembering that your body is not broken, your pleasure is valid, and your sexuality belongs to you.

You are in good hands.

Author's Note

This book is the convergence of personal curiosity and a professional calling.

As a somatic educator and integrative mental health practitioner, my work lives at the intersection of body and brain—bridging movement and mindfulness, science and sensuality.

Over the years, I've helped clients unravel how their nervous systems shape everything from stress and safety to pleasure, connection, and desire. One truth has become unmistakably clear: sexual vitality is not separate from our overall health—it is woven into the very fabric of our emotional and physical well-being.

Awaken Your Body, Awaken Your Desire was born from that understanding. It is the book I longed for—not just for my clients, but for my colleagues and for myself. A book that treats sexuality not as a problem to be fixed, but as a landscape to be explored. A book that honors evidence-based science and the lived wisdom of the body in equal measure.

This is not a manual for sexual "fixing." It's an invitation to presence. To notice what is already alive in you—and to deepen it. Through breath, movement, and mindful attention, we can create the inner conditions that allow desire to reemerge. We can understand how stress might be dimming that spark, and discover how to gently rekindle it.

If you've ever wondered whether pleasure could be intentional, whether science can serve eros, or whether your body holds more than just symptoms—you are not alone. This book is for you.

May these practices serve as a soft return to yourself: to sensation, to curiosity, to wholeness.

Thank you for being here. You are your own best guide—and I'm honored to walk beside you.

Now let's explore how to put this into practice.

Table of Contents

Before We Begin 1

Chapter 1: The Body Is the Way Back 7

Chapter 2: Is This You? 11

Chapter 3: The Hunt for What Actually Works 15

Chapter 4: It's Not You. It's the System. 19

Chapter 5: Where Science Meets Sensation 25

Chapter 6: Mapping the Body Back to Desire 29

Chapter 7: The Disconnect Was Never Your Fault 33

Chapter 8: The 6 Secrets That Change Everything 37

Chapter 9: Beyond Talk: The Science of Somatic Healing 51

Chapter 10: Self-Assessment: What's Happening in My Body? 59

Chapter 11: The Sexual Wellness Barriers 67

Chapter 12: Naming What You're Feeling 71

Chapter 13: The Quiet Barriers to Pleasure 89

Chapter 14: The Somatic Toolkit 101

    The Breathwork Techniques 103

    The Yoga Postures 133

    The Meditation Practices 199

Chapter 15: The Mindset Map 207

    The Journaling Practices 209

    Affirmations 220

Chapter 16: Healing Plans for the 14 Core Concerns 227

Chapter 17: Coming Home to Yourself 291

Trusted Clinical Resources 295

References 297

Before We Begin

If you've ever felt like something's missing from your sexual health journey, you're not alone.

For years, women have been told that issues with sexual intimacy, desire, or pleasure can be "fixed" with medication, talk therapy, or physical therapy. And while these approaches can offer relief, many women still find themselves asking:

- *Why don't I feel connected to my body?*
- *Why does sex feel mechanical—or even repelling—instead of pleasurable?*
- *What if nothing is actually broken... but I still don't feel like me?*

These are the questions that brought me here—and they might be what brought you, too.

Or maybe you're here because you've experienced pain, tension, or numbness during sex.

You may have been referred to pelvic floor therapy or given vaginal dilators. Many women are. And while some progress through the sizes, they're left wondering why desire and natural arousal haven't followed. I can't tell you how often I hear:

"*I did all the right things... and I still don't feel turned on.*"

That's because sexual health isn't just physical.

It's not just psychological.

It's *personal. Emotional. Energetic. Whole-body.*

Stress, emotions, and lived experiences don't just pass through us. They live in our tissues.

They shape how we feel, how we touch, and how we want—or don't want—to be touched.

That's where this book comes in.

Through somatic practices, breathwork, journaling, yoga, and mind-body techniques, you'll learn how to:

- Reconnect with your body and increase pleasure
- Release stored stress and tension
- Reframe long-held beliefs around sex, worth, and intimacy
- Reignite confidence and authentic desire—*on your terms*

You don't need to be fixed.

You just need to come home to yourself.

You may not need to spend years in therapy—whether that's psychotherapy or physical therapy, to reclaim your sexual well-being. While those approaches can offer support—and may even speed up the healing process for some—this book offers something different: a step-by-step, science-backed plan you can begin using today, right where you are.

A Note on Language

Throughout this book, you'll see me use terms like *"women"* and *"vulva-owners"* to honor the diverse range of people who may be navigating these challenges—regardless of gender identity, relationship status, or sexual orientation.

I know language can feel personal—and, at times, political. My aim is not to be clinical or distancing, but to speak with precision and care. Wherever you find yourself on the spectrum of gender or embodiment, please know this: you belong here.

You are seen. You are included. And this book was written with you in mind.

I'll also explain later why this kind of language matters—not just for inclusion, but for healing.

Your Roadmap for Using This Book

This isn't just another book about sexual health. It's an interactive guide meant to help you take action and see real results. Built around four simple steps, it walks you from self-awareness to meaningful, embodied transformation.

Step 1: Identify What You Need

Start with the self-assessment to explore which areas of your sexual wellness need the most care. Then turn to the chapters that speak directly to those concerns. These sections will give you the insight and context to understand what's showing up in your body.

Step 2: Select Your Healing Plan

Each healing plan is focused on a specific concern—like low desire, difficulty with arousal, or sexual pain. Once you've identified what's most relevant to you, go to the healing plan that fits. There's no need to research or overthink—each one is ready for you, step by step.

Step 3: Track Your Progress

Healing isn't about perfection. It's about showing up. Each plan weaves together daily tools like breathwork, yoga, journaling, meditation, and Cognitive Behavioral Therapy (CBT). Your job? Commit to the practice, not the outcome. Your journaling will serve as a practical tool for self-monitoring—helping you observe changes in mood, sensation, and how you relate to your body and experiences.

Step 4: Celebrate Your Transformation

As you move through the practices, you'll begin to notice meaningful shifts—in your body, your emotions, and your sense of connection. This book equips you with tools that aren't just powerful, but deeply personal: breathwork to regulate, yoga postures to reset, affirmations to rewire, and rituals to help you remember who you are. These aren't just techniques. They're invitations to come alive.

> Right now, you're on the edge of something sacred.
> You know the why. You've glimpsed the how.

> But before we begin, let me tell you what lives beneath these pages—
> The story behind the science.
> The truth inside the tools.

> This is where the work begins.
> And where I meet you—body to body, story to story.

By the way—if you're wondering what this all builds toward, you won't be left guessing. In Chapter 6, I'll show you a sample of the 30-day healing plan in full. It's gentle, step-by-step, and rooted in science—and it's designed to help your body shift from stress to sensation, from disconnect to desire.

For now, just know this: you're not reading for information alone. You're building toward transformation.

PART 1
COMING HOME TO YOUR BODY

Chapter 1

The Body Is the Way Back

Hi. Welcome.

I'm so glad you're here.

I'm Dr. Danielle—and this is where we begin.

I'm a licensed psychotherapist, clinical sexologist, and registered yoga teacher. This means I get to talk about feelings, desire, pleasure, and the body *all day long*. And honestly? I never get tired of it.

But the truth is, I didn't come to this work through textbooks or titles. I came to it through lived experience—my own, and the stories of countless women I've walked alongside for the past 15+ years.

Women who feel like something just isn't working when it comes to sex—desire that's gone missing, arousal that feels stuck, orgasms that never quite show up to the party, or pain that makes everything feel… complicated.

Women who've been told:
"Just relax."
"Have a glass of wine."
"Try harder."
Or—my personal favorite—"Maybe it's all in your head."

If any of that sounds familiar, friend, you're in the right place.

Because here's the truth:

Your body isn't working against you—it's been speaking the language of survival. Now it's time to help it speak the language of healing.

I wrote this book because I've seen too many brilliant, capable, caring women feel lost, ashamed, or just plain over it when it comes to intimacy. Many tell me they don't feel sexual. That it doesn't matter to them anymore. That maybe this is just how it is now.

But when we start working together—through breath, gentle movement, a little curiosity, and a whole lot of compassion—something begins to shift.

They realize:

Their body didn't forget how to *feel*. It just needed the right invitation.

Their body wasn't the problem. *It was the missing piece of the solution.*

With the right tools, I've watched women go from shut down to lit up—from "I think I'm broken" to "I didn't know I could feel this good."

And I want that for you.

This book offers what traditional sex therapy often leaves out: a practical, science-backed, body-based path to healing. It can serve as a powerful complement to your work with a therapist, or it can stand on its own as a guide. Either way, everything I share here is meant to support and deepen the healing you've already begun, are currently engaged in, or are courageously preparing to start. Whether you're struggling with low libido, difficulty getting turned on, pain, emotional walls, or simply a sense of disconnection.

In this book, you'll discover how to:
- Tune in to your body's cues and stop working against yourself
- Use breathwork and movement to open the door to pleasure
- Unlearn the unhelpful stories that keep you stuck and hold you back from intimacy
- Reclaim your confidence and feel more like *you*

You don't need to be "fixed."

You don't need to fake it.

You just need the right support—and maybe someone who believes in your body as much as I do.

I'm honored you're here. Let's get started (no glass of wine required).

Let This Be Your Permission Slip

If you're experiencing low desire, difficulty with arousal or orgasm, or pain during sex, please hear this:

You are not broken.

These experiences aren't signs of failure—they're often your nervous system's way of protecting you.

You'll hear this message repeated throughout the book. Not because I think you need convincing, but because beliefs shaped by stress, shame, and trauma take time to untangle. With gentle, consistent care, we can begin to replace those beliefs with something more honest:

Your body is *adaptable*.
Your body is *resilient*.
Your body is capable of *pleasure*.

This journey isn't about pushing yourself or performing a certain way. It's about coming home—to your body, your truth, and the parts of you that may have gone quiet in order to feel safe.

You'll be guided through practices that include somatic movement, breathwork, stillness, and journaling—tools grounded in research and shaped by real-world experience. These practices are meant to work together, gently and holistically.

Some of them may feel unfamiliar at first, especially if you're new to yoga, mindfulness, or body-based healing. That's okay. You don't have to do them perfectly—just stay curious. Let the process unfold as it is, not as you think it should be.

This work may challenge you. It's meant to.

But it's also built to support you.

So, if you're still here—if something inside you is whispering, *keep going*—then trust it.

You're exactly where you need to be.

Chapter 2

Is This You?

This book is for you if you've ever asked yourself:
- Why don't I feel desire the way I used to?
- Why does sex feel more like pressure than pleasure?
- Why won't my body respond, even when I *want* it to?
- Do I even enjoy sexual pleasure—on my own, or with someone else?
- Am I broken?

Let's start with what's most important: You are not broken.

Despite what you may have been taught, sexual wellness isn't just about hormones, attraction, or technique. It's about the relationship between your mind, your body, and your emotions—and how that relationship either sustains or disconnects.

When stress, trauma, self-doubt, or major life changes disrupt that connection, desire and pleasure don't just disappear.

They get buried—beneath layers of tension, exhaustion, and deeply held subconscious beliefs.

You're in the Right Place If...

No matter where you're starting from, if any of the following resonate—you belong here.

- You feel disconnected from desire and arousal.
  You want to want sex—but neither your mind nor your body seems to respond.

- You're struggling to feel good in your body.
  Whether it's low libido, pain, or a sense of disconnect, intimacy feels more like effort than ease.

- You've been told it's "all in your head" or to "just relax."
  But you know, deep down, there's more to the story.

- You have tried pelvic floor therapy.
  You may have used dilators, progressed through the sizes, even "graduated." But desire, arousal, and interest still feel out of reach—and no one helped you connect the dots.

- You've tried psychotherapy, medication, or waited for things to change.
  And yet, ease, excitement, and connection still feel far away.

- You're ready to take your healing into your own hands.
  You're not looking for a quick fix—you want lasting, embodied transformation.

If any of that sounds familiar, know this: you're not alone—and you're not out of options. This book offers a different kind of path—one grounded in science, shaped by the body, and built for real, lasting change. But first, let's get clear on what you won't find here.

Clarity is its own kind of intimacy—so let's name what this book isn't.

1. **It's not a one-size-fits-all solution.**
   Your sexuality is personal, and your healing should be too. This book helps you explore what works for *you*, not what's "supposed" to work.

2. **It's not a substitute for medical care.**

While the tools here are powerful, some conditions require medical attention. If something feels off physically, please trust yourself and seek expert support. I've included resources later in the book to help you find certified providers in your area.

3. **It's not about fixing you.**
   Because you're not broken. This book is about remembering who you are—by reconnecting with your body. It's about rebuilding your confidence. And it's about reclaiming what's yours: the pleasure and the power that never actually left you.

What This Journey Offers You

Here's what you can expect when you begin working with the healing plans in this book:

- A step-by-step path tailored to your unique needs and experiences
- A deeper connection with your body, your emotions, and the intimacy you have with yourself
- Proven techniques from sex therapy, somatic healing, and yoga—woven into daily, doable practices
- A renewed sense of confidence, self-trust, and the knowing that healing is possible

You deserve to feel good in your body.

You deserve pleasure, connection, and aliveness—not just with a partner, but within yourself.

Chapter 3

The Hunt for What Actually Works

You've just read that this book is different—and now you might be wondering: *How did I discover what really works?*

The truth is, I didn't stumble into this by accident. I went searching. Not casually. Not as a side project. But like a scientist obsessed with finding the missing piece of a puzzle. I threw myself into research, hands-on experience, and listening—deeply—to what my clients were saying.

I consulted with sexologists, pelvic floor therapists, medical doctors, and functional medicine practitioners. I dissected the research on stress, nervous system responses, blood flow, arousal, and pleasure. And the answer became strikingly clear: We were treating the mind, but ignoring the body or vice versa.

Because I'd seen the pattern: PT helped, but it didn't *fix* it. Talk therapy helped, but something still felt missing. Women would follow the protocols, do the exercises, show up for appointments… and still say, *"I've tried everything, but nothing really works."*

To reconnect the dots between function and feeling, we needed *movement* that spoke the body's language—gentle, curious, breath-infused.

Here's the thing — I can't stand a half-baked treatment plan. Healing isn't passive. It's not something that just *happens to you*. I've been a practicing psychotherapist since 2012, and if there's one thing I know for sure, it's this:

Real healing is active.

It takes intention, attention, and a whole lot more than just getting your steps in.

The Pattern Beneath the Problem

As a practitioner, I've worked in a wide range of settings—community mental health, hospitals, home health and hospice care, and eventually, private practice. I've had the privilege of sitting across from women of all ages, backgrounds, and belief systems. Over the years, I began to notice a pattern that cut across generations and diagnoses: women were exhausted. Not just physically, but emotionally, sexually, and spiritually.

I've collected data, yes—but more importantly, I've listened. I've seen firsthand how women take on countless roles as caregivers, partners, professionals, and leaders—often placing their own needs at the very bottom of the list. Sexuality becomes another item on the to-do list, rather than a source of joy, vitality, and connection. I've worked with women who weren't even seeking help for intimacy issues, yet underneath their anxiety, grief, or burnout, was a deep disconnection from themselves—and from pleasure.

What I've learned is this: when women aren't having fun in their lives, when they're not feeling playful, curious, or free in their bodies, their connection to desire fades. It doesn't happen all at once. It happens slowly—when caregiving crowds out curiosity, when schedules eclipse sensuality, when stress takes the place of self-prioritization.

That's not a personal failure. It's a cultural pattern. One that starts with how we're socialized to care about everything and everyone else first. But that pattern can be interrupted. This book is your invitation to make yourself a priority again—not performatively, but profoundly. Nourishingly. Lastingly.

Chapter 4

It's Not You. It's the System.

At first, I assumed the issue was non-compliance. Maybe my clients weren't following through with the recommendations. Maybe they were too impatient. Maybe they were hoping for a quick fix. But the more I listened—to my clients, to my colleagues, to the results we *weren't* getting—the clearer it became:

The problem wasn't the women.

The problem was the system.

For decades, sexual dysfunction in vulva-owners has been treated with the same standard tools: Cognitive Behavioral Therapy (CBT), medications, sex education, and pelvic floor physical therapy. And to be clear—each of these has value.

CBT can reframe the brain's thoughts around sex.

Medications may adjust key neurotransmitters and hormones.

Education helps fill in the gaps about how the body works.

Pelvic floor therapy can release chronic tension and improve circulation to areas essential for arousal and sensation.

They treat parts of the issue—thoughts, chemical messengers, muscles—but often ignore the embodied experience of pleasure, connection, and safety. They rarely address how trauma, stress, or numbness live in the nervous system. They don't offer a space to play, to feel, to explore. And they certainly don't teach women how to come back to themselves as whole, alive beings—not just patients or problems to solve.

That's why I began building a new framework—one that integrates your whole self—body, mind, and story—not just your symptoms.

Where the Traditional Tools Fall Short

Here's what no one wanted to say out loud:

For many people, the aforementioned approaches weren't enough.

Let's take a closer look.

Cognitive Behavioral Therapy (CBT) is one of the most well-established tools in mental health. It helps shift distorted thinking, reframe limiting beliefs, and improve emotion regulation. But in many cases, CBT is applied without a sexual health lens.

It focuses heavily on changing thoughts—which is helpful, yes—but not sufficient when the body itself is holding tension, trauma, or disconnection. CBT is valuable for shifting thoughts, but when the body is holding the story, mindset work alone can fall flat.

Real change requires more: nervous system regulation, body-based awareness, and the safety to truly feel.

In my experience, the issue isn't just faulty thinking. It's the stress, the performance pressure, and the deeply ingrained belief that "my body is broken." Thought patterns absolutely need support—but so does the body. Without practices like breathwork, somatic tracking, and body-based presence, the work remains stuck in the head. Reframing helps, but what women really need is to feel safe enough in their bodies to feel.

When therapy doesn't resolve things, medication is often the next suggestion. But it doesn't always bring the relief women hope for.

When women report pain, low desire, or symptoms that don't fit a neat diagnosis, they're too often handed a prescription—not a plan. Antidepressants may help with mood, but they frequently dull the very sensations women are trying to recover. I can't tell you how many times I've heard: "I already didn't feel much—and now I feel even less."

And while some medications—like hormone replacement therapy or estrogen creams—can play a supportive role at certain life stages, they're often offered without addressing the bigger picture. Too many women are told, "It's all in your head," and handed that script for an SSRI or anti-anxiety med. But they're not imagining things. Their bodies are speaking. They need someone who knows how to listen differently—with their whole presence, not just a prescription pad.

Again, without a full-body plan that includes stress reduction, arousal awareness, and pleasure pathways, medication alone often misses the mark. It helps the biological system, but doesn't necessarily rekindle connection.

Sex education is another piece of the puzzle, but let's be honest: most of us received sex ed that was fear-based, clinical, or nonexistent. As adults, the idea of taking a class on sex can feel intimidating or embarrassing. Many people end up turning to social media, porn, or books that promote a specific sexual modality like tantra—and while some of these sources offer insight, they don't always address the whole person or feel accessible in everyday life.

Pelvic floor physical therapy can be an essential part of healing—especially when pain, tension, or trauma is involved. The use of dilators to gently retrain the vaginal canal is often part of this work. But here's what most people don't say:

Pelvic floor PT is not sexual. It's not erotic. It's clinical. And that's how it should be.

Dilators are smooth plastic cylinders in various sizes—not sensual, just clinical. While they're vital for training the body to accommodate penetration, they don't do anything to awaken desire or spark erotic energy. Most physical therapists are focused on muscle coordination and pain reduction, not arousal or connection. That's exactly what they're trained for—and that's where their role ends.

This leaves many women with improved physical function—but no idea how to reintegrate that with feeling turned on. They're released from therapy, but most of the time no one shows them how to reconnect their body's new capabilities with their emotional, sensual, and sexual self.

That's where this book comes in.

We don't want to discard those methods. We don't want to replace the tools that help. We want to finish what they started. We want to fill in the gaps. Pairing mindset work with movement. Combining pelvic therapy with pleasure. Bringing the body back into the conversation—not as a problem to fix, but as a partner in healing.

That's why I created this new approach—one that blends science-backed techniques with emotional safety, sensual curiosity, and nervous system support. In this book, you're learning the component parts of how I built your healing plan from the ground up—one that doesn't just aim to fix a problem, but reconnects you with the pleasure, confidence, and joy that's been missing.

What Is Somatic Tracking?

If you're wondering what the heck I just mentioned—*somatic tracking*—let me explain. We'll go much deeper into this later, but I don't want to slide in terminology that leaves you hanging.

Somatic tracking is the practice of gently tuning in to your body's sensations—without judgment, pressure, or the need to fix anything.

It's a way of noticing what's happening inside (like tension, warmth, or numbness) and staying present with it, even if it feels unfamiliar.

This practice helps you build body awareness, reduce fear around sensation, and create safety in feeling. For many women and vulva-owners—especially those healing from stress, trauma, or disconnection—somatic tracking becomes a powerful way to reestablish trust with the body and slowly open the door to pleasure.

You don't have to do it perfectly. Just bring your attention, your breath, and a little curiosity. Let your body show you what it's holding—and what it's ready to release.

Chapter 5

Where Science Meets Sensation

When COVID first hit—when the world shut down almost overnight—uncertainty skyrocketed, and cortisol levels surged. In those early days of collective crisis, the women in my practice weren't just stressed—they were drenched in stress hormones. Suddenly, those who already tended to deprioritize themselves had to become everything to everyone: teacher, caretaker, therapist, crisis manager.

And do you know what tanks first when your body is stuck in fight-or-flight?

Desire. Arousal. Pleasure.
Stress chemicals smother bliss chemicals.

It's not a metaphor—it's neurochemistry. When your brain is flooded with cortisol and adrenaline, it deprioritizes dopamine, oxytocin, and other "feel-good" messengers that fuel desire, connection, and pleasure.

If we wanted to restore sexual function, we had to reverse the damage of chronic stress.

That's when it clicked—not just conceptually, but viscerally: The body wasn't a backdrop—it was the control center.

Every signal of stress, every whisper of arousal, every flicker of numbness—it all lived in the nervous system.

This wasn't just about the mind. It was physiology.

And if we wanted real change, the body couldn't be left out of the conversation—it had to lead it, from the inside out.

And the more I watched stress hijack sensation, the more urgent it became to find real tools—not just theories—for coming back into the body.

Evidence Meets Embodiment

I went to yoga teacher training in 2019—not because I wanted to chant or find my inner light, but because I needed a way to help my clients get out of their heads and into their bodies. I finished just a few months before the world shut down.

At the time, I didn't realize how essential those tools would become.

I wasn't looking for a new identity—I was looking for a bridge. A way to help women breathe into sensation, move in ways that supported circulation and arousal, and activate their parasympathetic nervous system—the one responsible for rest, safety, and connection.

It wasn't about yoga for yoga's sake. It was about physiology.

And what the research confirmed—and what I felt in my bones—was this: without embodiment, healing stays surface-level. It becomes cognitive, not cellular. Insight without integration. But when the body is invited in, the healing deepens. It roots. It lasts.

Magic Is Real—But So Is Physiology

Let's be clear: I am first and foremost a scientist. I'm a behaviorist. I don't buy into mystical claims when it comes to treatment. If something works, I need to understand *why* it works. If I'm going to tell my clients to roll out a yoga mat, I want the research to back it up. And the research? It was overwhelming.

Studies showed that yoga increased genital blood flow, reduced stress, enhanced interoception (the ability to sense internal bodily sensations), and improved sexual function. This wasn't a fluke—it was a *physiological* chain reaction that made perfect sense.

Now, don't get me wrong—I love the woo. My bookshelf has tarot decks. I burn palo santo. I believe in signs from the universe and that sometimes Mercury *really* is messing with your whole vibe. I'm the first one to light a candle on a new moon and pull an oracle card with my coffee.

But when it comes to healing—when it comes to pain, numbness, or disconnection from your own body—you need more than vibes. You need tools that work with your biology: your nervous system, your blood flow, your breath. You need a framework rooted in reality, not just moon cycles.

Because embodiment isn't a mood or a trend. It's not a necklace you wear or a filter you apply. It's a physiological experience—and when we honor that, healing becomes not only possible, but inevitable.

Chapter 6

Mapping the Body Back to Desire

D*esire isn't summoned by willpower—it's nurtured by safety, sensation, and self-connection.*

In the pages ahead, we'll weave the mystical and the measurable into a healing plan that speaks the language of your body—and invites you home to yourself.

I built this protocol to address the full spectrum of sexual concerns, blending evidence-based Western modalities with time-honored Eastern practices. Not because I suddenly became a yogi, but because the science made it impossible to ignore what had been missing: attunement to the self.

Some people will read this and assume I'm saying yoga is *the* answer. I'm not. I'm saying yoga is *part* of the answer. Someone whose pelvic floor is so tight they wince when they pee likely needs pelvic floor therapy. Someone consumed with anxiety around sex will benefit from CBT. These modalities aren't in competition—they're collaborators. What's needed is not a silver bullet, but a symphony of support.

They are complementary. They are an intricate collaboration.

Science Meets Stillness

And mindfulness? It's not about incense and 'Ommms' (ॐ) —though I'm not opposed to either. It's about retraining your brain to stay present in your body. It's about quieting the background noise of life long enough to notice what's actually happening inside you. It's learning to breathe through sensation instead of bracing against it.

If that sounds a little "woo," I get it. But here's the truth: it's also science. Like I said—I'm a sucker for the mystical. I let my oracle cards weigh in on big decisions, trust divine timing, and flirt shamelessly with synchronicity. But when it comes to healing pain, stress, or disconnection, we need tools grounded in physiology. We need practices that help us feel safe *in* our bodies, not just hopeful in our minds.

The Way Back to Yourself

So here we are: a training manual that blends biology, psychology, and embodied presence to help vulva-owners reclaim their sexual vitality. When I say "holistic," this is what I mean—a truly integrative path. Not just talk therapy. Not just prescriptions. Not just mindset shifts.

An actual, practical roadmap.

Because "just relax" wasn't working.
Because "try this pill" wasn't enough.
Because thinking differently about sex couldn't help if your body still felt unsafe to feel.

This is what works.
This is where the work gets personal—and powerful.

What It All Builds Toward: Your Daily Healing Plan

Before we go any further, let me show you where we're headed—because sometimes it helps to know what the destination looks like.

Mapping the Body Back to Desire

At the heart of this book is a step-by-step healing plan that takes just 27 minutes a day. It's gentle, science-backed, and intentionally designed to help your body shift from stress to safety, from shutdown to sensation.

Here's a sample of what one of these healing plans looks like:

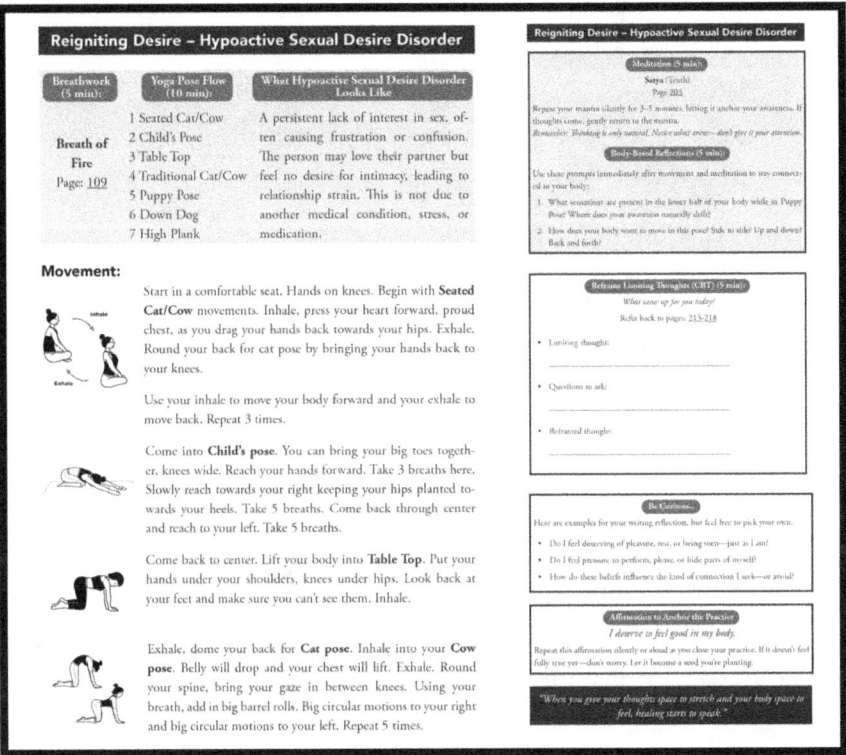

As you can see, it's already structured for you. No guesswork. Just follow the steps, and refer back to the chapters as needed for more detail or support.

Each daily session includes:

- **Breathwork:** 2–5 minutes
- **Yoga Postures:** 10–12 minutes
- **Meditation:** 3–5 minutes
- **Journaling:** 5 minutes

This combination invites your body into a regulated, receptive state where healing and desire can reawaken.

You'll also work with:

- **Cognitive Behavioral Therapy (CBT) tools** to gently challenge limiting beliefs about your body, sex, pleasure, and intimacy. These aren't required daily—just weekly reflections can create powerful change.
- **Affirmations** that act as quiet reinforcements. Pick one or two each week, post them where you'll see them, and update as needed. You'll know when it's time to shift.

And remember, this isn't about perfection.

It's about showing up.

These rituals aren't homework—they're invitations to come back to yourself, every day, in ways that feel doable and real.

This is the structure that thousands of women have used to reawaken their bodies—and I can't wait to walk you through it.

But before we begin the 30-day journey, there are a few more pieces we need to reclaim.

Specifically: the science, the language, and the truths you were never told about pleasure, anatomy, and desire.

Let's continue.

Chapter 7

The Disconnect Was Never Your Fault

Chances are, no one ever told you that stress and disconnection rewrite your body's response to pleasure. Or that your anatomy holds more power than the world ever gave it credit for.

This chapter is where we start to correct that.

Here, we name what's been left out—and why language, education, and biology matter more than you've been taught to believe.

"I Want to Want It, But I Just Don't"

Have you ever found yourself thinking:

- *"I love my partner, but I don't feel any desire."*
- *"I want to enjoy intimacy, but my body isn't responding."*
- *"It's like my sex drive is shut off, and I don't know why."*

If so, you're far from alone. In fact, it's incredibly common. And more importantly, having these kinds of thoughts doesn't mean you're broken, disordered, or doing anything wrong.

Desire isn't just about attraction. It's about what's happening inside your body—your stress levels, your hormones, your nervous system, your daily patterns. Most of us were never taught how chronic stress rewires our physiology, shutting down pleasure and connection. But here's the good news: it can be rewired.

This chapter is the start of the map to understand why your body feels the way it does—and how you can begin to change it.

Why No One Talks About This

Most of what we learn about sex—whether from school, media, or past partners—focuses on the mechanics, not the experience. We're told desire should be automatic, that intimacy should just happen, that arousal is a light switch.

But when it doesn't work that way, no one tells us why.

The truth? Sexual desire and our capacity for pleasure are deeply connected to stress, hormones, brain chemistry, and social conditioning. When those systems are off, it's not about being "dysfunctional"—it's about being human. The trouble is, we've never been taught how it all actually works.

That's where this book is different.

We're beginning to uncover some of the missing pieces: why so many women (or vulva-owners) feel disconnected from desire, why mainstream advice falls flat, and what you can do to finally feel something again.

The Vulva Is Not a Vagina

Why Getting It Right Unlocks More Pleasure

You've probably heard the terms *vulva* and *vagina* used interchangeably—but they're not the same thing. And that distinction matters, especially when it comes to pleasure.

The *vagina* is the internal canal. The *vulva*, on the other hand, includes the external genital anatomy: the labia majora, labia minora,

The Disconnect Was Never Your Fault

urethral opening, and clitoris—including its glans, hood, and internal crura (the legs). That last part? It's key.

The clitoris is the only organ in the human body designed solely for pleasure. It has no reproductive or urinary function—just pure sensation. People with penises don't have an equivalent.

And yet for generations, women have been told that penetration alone should be enough. Meanwhile, the most sensitive parts of their anatomy have been minimized, misunderstood, or completely left out of the conversation.

Language shapes what we pay attention to—and what we ignore. Reclaiming the word *vulva* isn't just anatomically correct. It's politically and personally powerful.

It's time to stop leaving pleasure out of the story.

It's time to stop expecting our bodies to respond to miseducation.

It's time to return to the full truth of our design.

Let's start calling things by their real names. That's where healing begins.

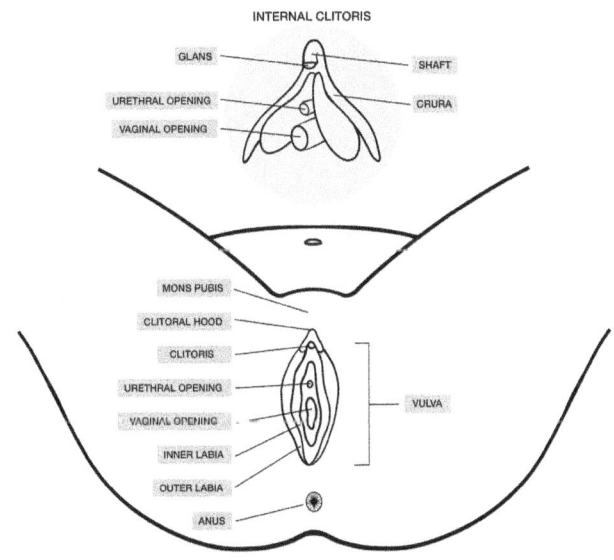

Chapter 8

The 6 Secrets That Change Everything

If you've ever wondered *why you feel the way you do*—or blamed yourself for not wanting sex—this chapter is for you.

These six truths will help reframe everything you thought you knew about desire.

They're not just secrets.

They're *clarity, chemistry, and reclamation*—and they'll change how you see your body, your pleasure, and your power.

Now let's get into the secrets.

These aren't just science facts—they're the missing links most people never learn.

Secret #1: Why Stress Kills Desire

"If my life is stressful, I just need to relax, right?"

Not quite.

Stress doesn't just make you "not in the mood"—it reshapes how your entire body functions. It dials down your ability to feel pleasure, to connect, to *want*.

Here's the truth: stress doesn't only live in your thoughts. It lives in your nervous system. And inside your body, there's a powerful command center that decides what matters most in any given moment. It's not trying to ruin your sex life—it's trying to keep you alive.

Let's talk about it.

The HPA Axis (Without A Lot of Science Jargon)

Deep in your brain and body, there's a system called the HPA Axis: your hypothalamus, pituitary gland, and adrenal glands. Together, they act like a traffic director for your energy and attention. Their job? To prioritize survival.

When your body perceives stress—whether it's a looming deadline, a tense relationship, or years of stored trauma—the HPA Axis kicks into high gear. It floods your system with stress hormones like cortisol and adrenaline, telling your body: *This is not the time for pleasure. This is the time to survive.*

Your heart races. Your digestion slows. Your muscles tense. Your arousal? Paused.

And it makes sense, right? If your body thinks you're under threat, the last thing it's going to do is open up to connection, softness, or sex.

But here's the good news: this system is adaptable. And with the right practices, you can teach your body that it's safe again. You can come down from the stress response and return to what I call your *pleasure physiology*—the state where desire naturally lives.

Meet Your Body's Stress Responders:

Part of the HPA Axis	Where It's Located	What It Does
Hypothalamus	In the lower middle part of the brain at the base of the brain, above the pituitary gland	Releases hormones for daily physiological cycles, controls appetite, regulates emotional responses, manages sex behavior, regulates body temperature

Pituitary gland	A pea-sized structure found at the base of the brain, behind the nose and inside the sella turcica	Secretes hormones for growth and sex/reproductive development and function, stimulates thyroid and adrenal glands plus the gonads, kidneys, uterus, and breasts
Adrenal glands	On top of each kidney, in the upper part of the abdomen. They are the size of a walnut	Produce hormones for metabolism, immune systems, blood pressure, and stress chemicals

Your HPA Axis is like your body's built-in stress alarm system. It constantly scans for threats and decides what's urgent… and what can wait.

Think of your brain like a smartphone. When too many apps are running, everything slows down. The HPA Axis chooses which "apps" to keep open during stress—and guess what?

Sex doesn't make the cut.

Here's what actually happens when your body is under stress:

1. Your brain picks up on the threat and sends out an emergency alert.
2. Your adrenal glands flood your body with cortisol (your main stress hormone).
3. Your nervous system shifts into survival mode: fight, flight, freeze, or fawn.
4. Your body powers down desire, pleasure, and connection—because they're not essential to survival.

And that's the key: if your brain thinks you're in danger, it doesn't care about intimacy or arousal.

It cares about keeping you alive.

This is why you can love your partner—and still feel no desire.

Your body isn't broken. It's doing exactly what it was designed to do.

It's choosing survival over sex.

Secret #2: How Social Media Is Hacking Your Pleasure System

"I just have a low libido."
"Maybe I'm just not built for pleasure."

Nope. Not true.
Your body was *designed* for pleasure.
But your brain? It's been hijacked.

Let's talk about dopamine—your pleasure and motivation chemical.

What Is Dopamine, Really?

Dopamine is like the engine of your desire—it drives you toward what feels good. It gives you that little "yes" feeling that says, *do that again.*
- Eat food you love? Dopamine hit.
- Hear a text ping? Dopamine hit.
- Get a "like" on social media? Dopamine spike.
- Have a beautiful, connected sexual experience? Another dopamine hit.

The problem isn't dopamine itself—it's what your brain learns to associate it with.

When your dopamine is constantly coming from your screen—scrolling, likes, texts, quick novelty—your brain starts to prefer fast, artificial stimulation over the slower build of real-world pleasure.

In other words: your reward system gets rewired.

Your brain starts to chase screen-based hits… and becomes less responsive to the richness of actual connection, intimacy, and embodied joy.

The Good News

This is reversible. You can retrain your brain. You can teach your body to crave depth over distraction.
With intention, you can shift from fragmented stimulation to full-bodied pleasure again.

Because your desire isn't broken.

It's just been redirected.

Secret #3: Arousal ≠ Desire

"I'm not turned on, so I must not want it… right?"
Not necessarily.

This is one of the most common myths I see in my practice—and one of the most damaging.

Desire and arousal are not the same.

They're separate processes in the body—and they don't always arrive at the same time.

Desire is the *interest* or the mental spark—the wanting.

Arousal is the *physical* response—blood flow, lubrication, nipple erection, genital swelling, that tingling aliveness.

You can have one without the other.

You might feel aroused without desiring sex (like during sleep, or in a medical exam).

And you can absolutely desire sex without immediately feeling aroused (like wanting closeness but your body feels slow to respond).

Here's the part no one teaches us:

For many women, arousal comes *after* you begin.

That's called responsive desire—a term first described by sex researcher Dr. Rosemary Basson—and it's completely normal.

Spontaneous vs. Responsive Desire

You've probably only ever heard about spontaneous desire—that lightning bolt feeling that shows up out of nowhere and makes you want to pounce.

That's real… but it's not the whole story.

Responsive desire is different.

It shows up *after* your body begins to feel safe, warm, connected, or engaged. After the first kiss. The cuddling. The massage. The fantasy. The moment of eye contact that softens something inside you.

It's like hunger:

- Spontaneous desire is a sudden craving.
- Responsive desire is when you start eating and realize—oh wow, I was hungry after all.

Why This Changes Everything

If you're waiting to feel turned on before you touch yourself, connect with your partner, or initiate intimacy… you might be waiting forever.

Responsive desire doesn't mean there's something wrong with you. It means you're human.

Your body might just need space, time, and safety to get on board.

The takeaway?

If arousal doesn't come first, it doesn't mean desire isn't there.

Sometimes, you have to begin… and let your body catch up.

Secret #4: Outercourse Isn't Optional—It's How Our Bodies Work

Let's talk about something most women were never taught: how your body actually gets turned on.

Here's what you probably *didn't* learn in sex ed:

- Most vulva-owners need 20 to 45 minutes to become fully aroused
- Outercourse isn't just a warm-up—it's the primary pathway to arousal *and* pleasure for vulvas for the whole experience, start to finish
- And penetration? That's only the "main event" if *you* want it to be

These aren't just opinions—they're backed by decades of sex research on female sexual response. But no one taught us this.

A Quick Word on Foreplay

Let me be blunt: what many people call "foreplay" is not a warm-up—it's often the *whole damn show*. And not only that, stimulation to the vulva, especially the clitoris, will totally change the sensory experience if you do want penetration too. For the better. Ohhh, the pleasure.

Manual stimulation, oral sex, toys, fantasy, massage, breathwork—this is sex if it brings you into your body and into pleasure.

For men, foreplay often enhances pleasure.

For most women, it's a necessity for them to have the utmost pleasure. The pleasure that increases your interest in being sexual more often. To me, that's a win for everyone.

So, it's time to retire the idea that real sex = penetration. Outercourse isn't optional.

Quick tip: Use a small handheld vibrator during penetration if you're having sex with a penis. It's not a competitor to your partner, it's a collaborator. You'll thank me later, I promise.

You're Not Broken—You're Just Rushed

When you don't know how long arousal takes—or that your body blooms in waves, not lightning bolts—it's easy to believe something is wrong.

"I must not be into this."
"I'm broken."
"I have low libido."

But the truth?

You're not broken.
You've just been rushed.
You have a body that needs time, the right kind of touch—and time to *build up* before you go over the edge.

Secret #5: The Lie That's Keeping You Stuck in a Sex Rut

"But we used to have sex all the time when we first got together."
Sound familiar?

It's one of the most common refrains I hear from partners—and one of the biggest misunderstandings about desire in long-term relationships.

It's not malicious. It's not even wrong… it's just incomplete.

The Truth About New Relationship Energy

In the early days of love, your brain is riding high on a potent cocktail of bliss chemicals:
- Dopamine from novelty
- Oxytocin from bonding

Mix in the *mystery* that heightens attention and arousal, and you've got the perfect conditions for "effortless" desire.

This phase of intensity is often called *new relationship energy*—and it's why spontaneous desire felt so easy in the beginning.

But over time, things shift.
The relationship stabilizes.
Your brain settles into safety and routine.

Which is good for your nervous system… but harder on "instant" arousal.

You're not less attracted to your partner.
You're just in a different phase—one that asks for presence instead of novelty.

So, What Changed?

You haven't lost desire.
You've lost differentiation—the sense of otherness, tension (the good kind), and mystery that naturally fuels erotic charge.

And that's okay. It doesn't mean something's broken. It just means desire needs a new kind of fuel.

The Fix? Body-Based Aliveness

When things feel stuck or stale, the answer isn't to "try harder." It's to get out of your head—and back into your body.

You don't need to force intimacy.
(Though scheduling sex? Can be HOT. Who doesn't want to build a little anticipation?)

What you really need is to reawaken your own sensual system—through movement that feels good, creativity that energizes you (the kind that invites embodiment and emotional expression), nervous system practices that bring calm, and a renewed intimacy with your own body and pleasure.

Because you can't manufacture desire.
But you *can* create the conditions where it returns.

Secret #6: The One Thing That Keeps You Connected & Blissful

(Hint: It's the thread that ties your healing together.)

The secret?

Movement.

Not punishment.
Not perfection.
Not hitting a number or tracking a goal.

I'm talking about intentional, sensual, soul-guided movement—designed to wake up your nervous system, soften your body's defenses, and reconnect you with your pleasure.

Why Movement Changes Everything

Science tells us what your body already knows:

- **Movement reduces cortisol**, your body's primary stress hormone—lowering inflammation, anxiety, and emotional reactivity
- **It increases endorphins**, natural opioids that elevate mood, reduce pain, and enhance overall well-being
- **It supports hormonal regulation**, including estrogen and testosterone levels tied to desire, arousal, and mood stability
- **It stimulates the vagus nerve**, enhancing parasympathetic tone—critical for shifting out of fight-or-flight and into states of safety, trust, and sexual receptivity
- **It improves blood flow**, especially to the pelvic region—supporting genital arousal, lubrication, and heightened sensation

In other words: movement restores your connection to your body. And in your body, desire begins to awaken.

What Kind of Movement?

It's not about "working out." It's about working *in*.

- Breathwork that calms your system and turns numbness into presence
- Yoga that rewires your body for safety and sensation
- Stretching that melts tension and reawakens pelvic vitality
- Dancing that shakes off shame and brings you back to joy *(okay, not officially in your plan—but you should absolutely do it)*

These are not extras.
These are your reconnection rituals.

Pleasure Is a Practice

This book isn't just a guide—it's an invitation.
To come back into rhythm with yourself.
To feel what you feel.
To move what's been stuck.
To remember that desire isn't out there waiting for the right moment or the right person or the right spark.

It's already inside you.
Movement is the key that unlocks it.

And maybe eventually we can add another movement bullet to that list above:

- Sex as movement—rhythmic, attuned, and rooted in pleasure and trust

The 6 Secrets Are Yours: To Keep or To Share

You've just uncovered the six secrets—
not to fix your desire, but to finally understand it.
Not to force your body, but to come back to it.

Because maybe it's not that your desire is gone.

Maybe it's been quiet, waiting for the right conditions to rise again.

Waiting for softness instead of pressure.

For truth instead of performance.

For movement, breath, safety, and slowness.

Your body remembers.

Even when your mind forgets.

These secrets aren't just ideas.

They're invitations.

To return.

To feel.

To begin again—with your body, your pleasure, your pace.

Let this be the moment you stop chasing desire…

and start creating the world it wants to come home to.

PART 2
RECLAIMING PLEASURE THROUGH AWARENESS & UNDERSTANDING

Chapter 9

Beyond Talk: The Science of Somatic Healing

Across these last chapters, you've been reorienting—seeing desire, stress, and sensuality through the lens of embodiment, not dysfunction.

Now we shift from hearing about your body to understanding what it's trying to say.

Before we dive into your healing plan, we need clarity: how stress, trauma, and physiology have shaped your pleasure—and what your body is asking for now.

You'll explore the somatic roots of sexual healing.

You'll practice noticing what's happening inside—without shame, without blame.

And you'll gather tools to help your nervous system feel safe enough to repair, reconnect, and respond.

You're not just preparing for the work ahead.

You're doing it—right here, by learning to listen.

What is Somatic Therapy?

If you're wondering what somatic therapy is, let me save you a Google search:

It's the practice of treating emotional pain through the body.

Trauma, stress, and emotion don't just live in your mind—they live in your tissues, your breath, your posture.

If your stomach has ever dropped from anxiety, or your shoulders tensed during stress, you already know what I mean.

Traditional talk therapy is helpful—but it mostly works from the neck up.

Somatic therapy works from the inside out.

It helps you reconnect with physical sensation and use breath, movement, and awareness to process what's stuck.

It's not just insight—it's integration.

And for women facing sexual disconnection, shutdown, or pain, this is essential.

Because you can't think your way into desire.

You have to feel your way into it.

The Deeper Roots of Mindfulness

In an earlier chapter, we began exploring mindfulness as a tool for reconnecting with your body. Now, let's go deeper—because a lot of people assume mindfulness is some trendy, mystical, or even "woo-woo" idea.
Spoiler: it's not.

Yes, mindfulness is deeply rooted in Buddhist and Hindu traditions—but that's not the whole story.

It also shows up across many spiritual lineages, including Judaism, Christianity, and Islamic traditions.

In Jewish traditions, meditative prayer and embodied reflection have existed for centuries.

Christian mystics practiced what they called *centering prayer*—a quieting of the mind to connect with the divine.

In Islamic traditions, *dhikr* is a rhythmic repetition of sacred words to foster presence and inner calm.

So, if you've ever worried that mindfulness might conflict with your beliefs or feel unfamiliar—take a deep breath.

This is not a foreign practice.

It's a human one.

At its core, mindfulness is the practice of being here.

Fully present.

Fully in your body.

Fully in the moment.

And if you're struggling with desire, pleasure, or connection, this skill will become one of your greatest allies.

Mindfulness in Western Psychology: The Science Behind It

Mindfulness first gained mainstream recognition in Western psychology thanks to Jon Kabat-Zinn, who developed the Mindfulness-Based Stress Reduction (MBSR) program in the late 1970s at the University of Massachusetts Medical School.

His 8-week program was designed to reduce stress and improve physical and emotional well-being—and it worked. The outcomes were so promising that MBSR became the foundation for other clinical approaches, including Mindfulness-Based Cognitive Therapy (MBCT), a treatment specifically designed for preventing relapse in Major Depressive Disorder.

Around the same time, in 1975, the Insight Meditation Society was founded by Jack Kornfield, Sharon Salzberg, and Joseph Goldstein. They helped bring meditation and mindfulness practices into the American mainstream, blending ancient wisdom with psychological insight—and making these tools more accessible for both clinicians and the general public.

As evidence grew, psychology began to fully embrace mindfulness. Research confirmed its effectiveness in treating depression, anxiety, chronic stress, and even trauma. Today, mindfulness is woven into many of the most effective evidence-based therapies, including Acceptance and Commitment Therapy (ACT) and Dialectical Behavior Therapy (DBT).

The takeaway?

Mindfulness isn't just an ancient spiritual practice.

It's a scientifically validated tool—and it's one we'll be using in this book in a way that's practical, embodied, and specifically tailored to support your sexual healing.

Why These Healing Tools?

You're doing the unlearning. Now it's time to add in the return—the rebirth. These are the tools that will support your healing—practices that meet your body where it is, and gently invite it into something new.

This book can't just give you information.

It has to give you a process.

You're not here to read about sex healing.

You're here to live it—to feel it in your body, and to begin the kind of transformation that actually lasts.

The tools you'll be working with aren't random. They're carefully chosen to do three very specific things:

- Calm your nervous system
- Reconnect you with your body
- Retrain your brain to experience pleasure

Here's what you'll be practicing and why:

- **Breathwork** – Calms the nervous system, increases oxygen flow, and grounds you in the present
- **Gentle Yoga movements** – Improve circulation, increase flexibility, and support pelvic awareness and vitality
- **Meditation** – Build awareness, presence, and a deeper relationship with your body
- **Journaling prompts** – Help you explore emotions, beliefs, and patterns that may be blocking pleasure
- **CBT-based reframing exercises** – Shift the negative thoughts you may hold about sex, your body, or connection
- **Affirmations** – Support subconscious healing and invite self-compassion

Each of these practices is a pathway back to yourself.

They're designed to help you listen, soften, and gently rewire your nervous system to feel safe enough for connection—and regulated enough to access pleasure without overwhelm.

The Goal: Sensual Awareness, Not Just Sex

Let's be clear: this isn't about revving up your sexual energy just for the sake of it.

This is about sensual awareness.

Before you can feel pleasure with someone else, you need to feel it within yourself.

That starts by waking up your senses, finding your own rhythm, and tuning into the subtleties of what your body wants.

We're not here to force desire. That backfires.

What works is regulating the nervous system, developing self-attunement, and supporting your body's natural production of feel-good neurochemicals—like dopamine and serotonin.

These are the same chemicals that support motivation, elevate your mood, and create that quiet, grounded vitality where pleasure becomes possible.

And when you do connect with someone else?

You get the added support of oxytocin, the "love hormone" that deepens trust, intimacy, and satisfaction.

But here's the best part:

You don't have to wait for someone else to generate these states.

You can cultivate them from within.

Through consistent, body-based practices, you begin to rewire how you experience safety, connection, and sensual joy.

Sex, pleasure, and desire don't need to be achieved.

They emerge naturally—when you start feeling good again.

And when you feel better, you connect more.

With your body. With your desire. And with whatever (or whoever) you want to welcome in.

The Plan: 30 Days of Practice

For the next 30 days, you'll follow a structured, science-backed process—one that gently reconnects you with your body, rewires stress patterns, and invites your desire to come home. You saw a similar list above, but let me show you once more, with descriptions of what you'll be doing. I don't know about you, but I need to keep seeing, keep hearing, and keep imagining, so that I feel prepared before I take on anything new or unfamiliar.

Each day, you'll move through six core practices:

1. **Breathwork** – Simple, guided breathing exercises to calm your nervous system and bring you into the moment
2. **Yoga postures** – A beginner-friendly targeted sequence or flow (equally wonderful for experienced yogi's)
3. **Journaling prompts** – Thoughtfully crafted questions to help you explore what you were feeling in your body or thinking in your mind
4. **CBT-based exercises** – Tools to shift negative thought patterns about sex, your body, or connection
5. **Meditation** – Short, focused moments of stillness using a specific mantra
6. **Affirmations** – Daily intentions to repeat or post for your brain to passively see

These aren't random.

The order matters.

The repetition matters.

This sequence is intentionally designed to regulate your nervous system, re-pattern your response to pleasure, and create lasting, embodied change.

So, here's the deal:

Follow the process. Show up for yourself. Do the work—even when it's uncomfortable, even when it's inconvenient.

You've tried all the things—fixes, hacks, pressure, self-blame.

Now it's time to try something different.

Something that actually connects your mind *and* body in a way that makes sense—because it's how you're actually wired to heal.

A Pause for Honest Self-Assessment

By now, you've got the framework.

You understand the tools—and how they work together to bring your body back into connection, safety, and pleasure.

But before we leap into your personal 30-day plan, I want you to pause.

Not because you're not ready.

But because clarity is powerful.

This isn't a one-size-fits-all journey.

And the truth is, your body may be holding specific stress patterns or sexual health concerns that deserve thoughtful attention.

So, before we move on to the *how*, let's get clear on the *what*.

Let's listen to your body—and let it show us where to go.

Now that you know what the plan looks like, let's make sure it's the *right* plan—for you.

Chapter 10

Self-Assessment: What's Happening in My Body?

If you've been struggling with your body, your desire, or your ability to feel pleasure, you may have asked yourself:

What's wrong with me?

Let's clear this up right now: you are not broken.

Yes, I've said it before. Fourteen times, actually.

And I'll keep saying it. Roll your eyes if you must—but I want this to sink in.

Your body isn't betraying you—it's communicating with you.

But if no one ever taught you how to read those signals, it's easy to misinterpret them as failure. They're not failure.

They're *information*.

This chapter is about understanding what your body's been trying to say.

We'll explore two key areas:

1. **The Stress Factor** – Is your body stuck in stress mode? What's it doing to your nervous system, your hormones, and your access to pleasure?

2. **The Sexual Health Factor** – Are there specific concerns affecting your arousal, desire, or comfort—and how can you begin to address them?

This is your chance to take stock—with zero shame and total clarity. Let's listen in.

Part A: Is Stress Running the Show?

Most people know that stress is bad for them. But what they don't always realize is that chronic stress rewires the body and brain in ways that directly impact everything from mood to immune function—and yes, even sexual desire.

Your nervous system is designed to move fluidly between two states:

- **Sympathetic mode** – Often called "fight-or-flight," this stress response kicks in when your brain perceives a threat. Heart rate increases, digestion slows, muscles tense, and your body floods with cortisol and adrenaline to help you respond quickly. This is crucial for short-term survival—but not sustainable long-term.

- **Parasympathetic mode** – Known as "rest-and-digest" or even "feed-and-breed," this is the state where healing, relaxation, emotional connection, and sexual arousal happen. It's regulated by the vagus nerve and is essential for hormone balance, immune function, and pleasure.

Your nervous system is like a light switch: when you're racing to meet a deadline, arguing with a partner, or scrolling bad news at midnight, your system flips into sympathetic mode. But if the switch gets stuck there, your body never gets the healing, connecting, or resetting time it desperately needs.

Self-Assessment: What's Happening in My Body?

If your body is stuck in stress mode, it doesn't just affect your mood—it impacts your hormones, your circulation, your muscle tension, and even your ability to feel aroused.

Common Signs That Your Body is in Chronic Stress Mode

Below is a list of some of the messages your body may be sending when it's stuck in fight-or-flight mode:
- Feeling overwhelmed or anxious most of the time
- Constant fatigue, even after sleeping
- Frequent headaches or migraines
- Digestive issues (bloating, IBS, acid reflux)
- Muscle tension, especially in the neck, shoulders, or jaw
- Racing thoughts or trouble focusing
- Increased or decreased appetite
- Mood swings or frequent irritability
- Trouble feeling connected to your own body

Sound familiar?

If so, don't stop at "Yes, I'm stressed."

Ask yourself:

Has my body forgotten how to return to safety and calm?

What are my stress symptoms trying to tell me?

The Long-Term Effects of Chronic Stress

If your nervous system stays in survival mode for too long, your body forgets how to regulate itself. That's when deeper health issues start to surface—many of which get misdiagnosed or medicated without ever addressing the root cause: *nervous system dysregulation.*

Here are some of the conditions that can be triggered or worsened by chronic stress:
- Autoimmune diseases (Lupus, rheumatoid arthritis, MS)
- Hypertension (High blood pressure)

- Affective disorders (Mood disorders)
- Major depression
- Generalized anxiety disorder
- IBS and other gut disorders
- Chronic fatigue syndrome
- Adrenal dysfunction
- Sexual dysfunction (low desire, pain, or arousal issues)
- Altered sleep patterns (difficulty falling or staying asleep)
- Waking up frequently during the night
- Food cravings (especially for sugar and carbs)
- Weight fluctuations (gaining or losing without a clear cause)
- Low motivation to move or exercise
- Feeling emotionally numb or disconnected
- Brain fog or forgetfulness
- Frequent colds or low immunity

This isn't about diagnosing yourself.

It's about recognizing patterns.

If you see yourself in multiple categories above, your body might be waving a white flag, telling you that it's time to reset your nervous system and shift back into a healing state.

How many of the above-listed items are you experiencing?

The higher the number, the more likely it is that your stress levels have reached the point of chronic stress.

But know this:

You're not doomed. You're just depleted.

You don't need to be fixed—you need to be refueled.

You need the right tools, the right context, the right support.

Self-Assessment: What's Happening in My Body?

Part B. Understanding Your Sexual Health

Sexual concerns are often brushed off as "all in your head."

But if something isn't working the way you want it to, it's real.

To help you understand what might be happening, I've created a friendly, easy-to-follow self-assessment—adapted from the DSM-5 diagnostic criteria—to give you clarity on what's going on with your sexual function.

Take your time answering these questions.

Be honest with yourself.

There are no wrong answers.

Self-Assessment Quiz: Understanding Your Sexual Health

1. Do you rarely or never feel interest in sex, even though you once did?
2. Do you feel interested in sex, but experience little to no physical arousal?
3. Do you feel intense fear, disgust, or avoidance toward sexual activity?
4. Do you struggle with uncontrollable sexual urges or behaviors?
5. Do you find it difficult or impossible to orgasm?
6. Do you experience pain during penetration?
7. Do your vaginal muscles involuntarily tighten, making penetration painful or impossible?
8. Are you postmenopausal and experiencing vaginal dryness or discomfort during sex?
9. Do you have chronic vulvar pain, burning, or irritation that happens outside of sex as well?
10. Do you experience deep pelvic pain, especially around your menstrual cycle, or feel a sharp internal pain during penetration?

If more than one of these feels familiar, don't worry—you may want to explore a few different sections in this book.

Knowledge is power—and now, you have it.

Note which questions you answered yes to.

This isn't about labeling yourself—it's about getting clear on what's asking for support.

If these words feel a little cold and clinical, don't worry. We're about to warm them up—wrap them in stories, sensations, and the tender edges of real-life intimacy, where the heart of these struggles truly begins to make sense. But first, let's take a quick look at the key.

Key to Sexual Health Concerns

Let's be clear: you don't have all of the conditions listed below.
And the good news? There aren't dozens of confusing possibilities. In fact, there are just 10 primary sexual concerns for vulva owners—and this book addresses every one.

Each numbered question above corresponds to a numbered condition below.

So if you answered "yes" to #3, take a look at #3 in this list.

(And just so you know—you only need to read the one that fits your experience.)

1. **Hypoactive Sexual Desire Disorder (HSDD)** – Persistent lack of sexual interest or desire
2. **Sexual Arousal Disorder (SArD)** – Difficulty achieving physical arousal despite interest
3. **Sexual Aversion Disorder (SAvD)** – Strong negative reactions to sexual activity, including fear or disgust
4. **Hypersexuality / Compulsive Sexual Behavior (HCSB)** – Inability to control sexual thoughts or behaviors
5. **Anorgasmia** – Inability or difficulty reaching orgasm

Self-Assessment: What's Happening in My Body?

6. **Dyspareunia** – Pain during penetration that isn't caused by another medical condition
7. **Vaginismus** – Involuntary tightening of vaginal muscles, making penetration painful or impossible
8. **Vaginal Atrophy** – Postmenopausal thinning and dryness of vaginal tissue, leading to discomfort
9. **Vulvodynia** – Chronic vulvar pain, burning, or irritation with no clear cause
10. **Endometriosis** – Deep pelvic pain, especially around your menstrual cycle or a sharp internal pain during penetration

What Comes Next?

Now that you have a clearer picture of what's happening in your body, it's time to take action.

This book is designed to guide you through the next steps:

- If stress is running the show, you'll learn how to shift into healing mode
- If a sexual health issue resonates with you, you'll explore gentle, body-based tools to support healing

But most importantly?

You're learning to work *with* your body—not against it.

Let's keep going.

Chapter 11

The Sexual Wellness Barriers

It's coming into focus now—the shape of what's really going on. Sexual disconnection isn't just in your head. It lives in your body, your past, your nervous system. And it's more common than you've been led to believe.

In this chapter, we name the most common roadblocks to sexual vitality and offer a practical way forward. These aren't just diagnoses—they're patterns. And by naming them, we begin to reclaim our power.

The 10 Most Common Barriers to Sexual Wellness

For clarity, I've grouped the 10 most common concerns into four categories, using both clinical language and plain terms you can actually relate to:

1. *Sexual Desire Disorder*

- **Hypoactive Sexual Desire Disorder (HSDD):** A persistent lack of sexual desire that feels distressing.

2. *Sexual Arousal Disorders*

- **Sexual Arousal Disorder:** You want to feel aroused but your body isn't responding.
- **Sexual Aversion Disorder:** You experience strong discomfort, fear, or disgust toward sexual contact.

- **Hypersexuality / Compulsive Sexual Behavior**: You feel out of control with your sexual thoughts or behaviors.

3. *Orgasmic Disorder*
    - **Anorgasmia**: You find it difficult or impossible to reach orgasm.

4. *Sexual Pain Disorders (a.k.a. Penetration Disorders)*
    - **Dyspareunia**: Pain during intercourse or penetration.
    - **Vaginismus**: Involuntary tightening of the vaginal muscles.
    - **Vaginal Atrophy**: Dryness and fragility, especially after menopause.
    - **Vulvodynia**: Chronic vulvar pain or irritation with no clear cause.
    - **Endometriosis / Pelvic Adhesions**: Deep internal pain, often linked to menstrual cycles or scar tissue.

But That's Not the Whole Picture...

Beyond these diagnoses, there are four emotional and psychological blocks I see over and over again in my work with women:

- **Low Self-Esteem**
- **Poor Body Image**
- **Struggles with Self-Love**
- **Unrecognized (or Unspoken) Trauma**

These are not lesser concerns. They are deeply woven into how we experience sexuality—and they deserve just as much attention.

That's why each of these has its own healing plan in this book. You can follow a plan for one of the clinical concerns *and* add one of these emotional healing tracks to support your full self.

How It All Comes Together: A Real-Life Example

Let's look at how this works in practice.

The Sexual Wellness Barriers

Meet Kate.
After completing the self-assessment, Kate realized she was experiencing anorgasmia. She didn't identify with any of the emotional healing tracks—so she chose to focus solely on the plan for orgasmic difficulty.

She read the chapter on anorgasmia (up next), then visited the section on unhelpful thinking patterns to challenge her beliefs about her body and pleasure. She chose a consistent time in the morning to do her daily practice, and set up a small, inviting space to move, breathe, and reflect.

In the beginning, her sessions took 35 minutes. By week two, she had eased into the rhythm—completing each day in 27 minutes or less. After about 10 days, she noticed she felt more at ease in her body. Soon, she was showing up differently with her partner—more open, more confident, more connected.

"It all started to come together," Kate shared. "It didn't feel forced. It felt… natural. Like I was finally doing what my body needed."

Your Plan Is Customizable—and Already Built

Each healing plan in this book includes a full 30-day protocol. You don't need to figure it out from scratch. Simply turn to the plan that matches your needs and follow along.

Each one draws from the same toolkit—breathwork, movement, meditation, and journaling—but the focus shifts depending on your specific concern.

You're about to see the healing plan formula again.

I know I've shown it to you a couple of times already—that's on purpose.

Repetition is a form of care. It's how the body learns safety. Patterns build trust.

So if it feels repetitive, good. Let it.

The more you see the rhythm, the more your system knows what to expect—and what to soften into.

Remember, your plan includes:
1. Breathwork to regulate the autonomic nervous system and support parasympathetic activation
2. Targeted yoga postures to increase interoceptive awareness and support somatic integration
3. Meditation to promote neural pathways of safety, openness, and self-attunement
4. Journaling and CBT-based prompts to identify and restructure unhelpful beliefs
5. Affirmations to reinforce adaptive thought patterns and embodied self-trust

You'll also find a "cheat sheet" in each plan for quick reference—full details are provided in the corresponding chapters.

Where to Next?

Next, we'll meet the sexual wellness barriers one by one—exploring what they are, how they feel, and eventually how to work with them gently and effectively.

This is not about labeling yourself.

It's about understanding your body's signals—so you can respond with care.

Now that you know what you're working with, you're ready to dive deeper—into each barrier, and into your own healing.

Chapter 12

Naming What You're Feeling

Understanding the real meaning behind common sexual struggles —without the clinical coldness.

In this chapter, we'll take a closer look at some of the most common sexual challenges vulva-owners face.

These are often referred to as "disorders" in the medical world—but here, we approach them differently. That's why you're seeing me use words like "sexual wellness barriers," "sexual challenges," and "roadblocks." We're not labeling you—we're equipping you. Because when you understand what's really going on in your body and mind, you can move forward with clarity, confidence, and a plan that actually meets you where you are.

What follows is a plain-language breakdown of what each condition actually means, how it might show up in real life, and how you can start working with it—rather than against it.

Anorgasmia

When the peak doesn't come—and you're left wondering why.

Let's talk about orgasm. Or more specifically—what happens when it's delayed, elusive, or completely absent.

If you're feeling turned on, receiving the kind of touch that *should* lead to orgasm—especially around the clitoris, your body's epicenter of pleasure—but the release still doesn't come… you might be navigating anorgasmia.

You are not alone. This is more common than most people realize.

For some, orgasm has always felt out of reach. For others, it used to be possible—but faded over time, maybe after childbirth, a trauma, or an overwhelming season of stress. Some can orgasm solo but not with a partner. Others find that pleasure builds… but never quite crests. And some experience no release at all, no matter the context.

Remember: for most vulva-owners, orgasm isn't a happy accident. It's the result of clear, consistent clitoral stimulation—usually through outercourse, not penetration. This isn't a failure of your body. It's a failure of what you were (or weren't) taught.

So, what's going on?

There are many potential contributors, including:

- A history of sexual or emotional abuse
- A lack of understanding around your own pleasure
- Struggles with body image or performance anxiety
- Guilt, shame, or pressure around sex
- Cultural or religious conditioning that makes pleasure feel "wrong"
- Ongoing life stress that disconnects you from your body
- Mental health factors like anxiety or depression
- Worry about your partner's feelings—or difficulty communicating your needs

If any of that sounds familiar, take a breath.

You're not broken. You're not failing. You're responding.

And now you have a name for it—and that's where healing begins.

This plan isn't about "trying harder" or forcing your body to perform.

It's about creating the safety, clarity, and slowness your pleasure needs to unfold.

Step by step, you'll learn to reconnect with sensation, release pressure, and reawaken orgasm from the inside out.

Hypersexuality/Compulsive Sexual Behavior

When desire becomes a compulsion—and it stops feeling like choice.

Let's kill the myth: this is not *sex addiction.*

That term isn't real—at least not clinically. It's not recognized by the DSM. It's not accepted by the American Association of Sexuality Educators, Counselors and Therapists (AASECT), which is also the organization I'm certified through. While some clinicians still use the label 'sex addiction,' it often misses the mark—and can turn into a shame stick instead of a helpful diagnosis.

Here's what *is* real:

You can have a healthy sex drive and still feel out of control.

You can crave sex—and still feel trapped by the way you're using it.

You can be functional in life—but your browser history, your patterns, and your emotions tell a different story.

This is hypersexuality. And it's not about wanting sex.

It's about needing it to numb something deeper.

It becomes compulsive. You think about it constantly. You chase the high. You feel that internal itch and scratch it in ways that don't feel good later. Not because you're broken—but because somewhere along the line, this became your coping strategy.

It's not the sex that's the problem.

It's what the sex is standing in for.

You might be navigating hypersexual behavior if:

- You tell yourself you'll stop—then don't
- You feel "gross" after, but keep going back
- You get defensive when anyone brings it up
- You lie about it, hide it, or downplay it
- You use it to calm down, check out, or feel "enough" for five damn minutes
- You've burned through relationships or trust because of it

This is where desire crosses the line into compulsion. Not because you're bad. Not because you're "too much." But because you're human—and this is how you've learned to soothe.

The good news?

This pattern is unlearnable. Your true desire can be reclaimed.

But it begins with honesty—and a willingness to feel what's underneath the urge.

That's where this plan comes in.

You'll learn how to ground your nervous system, interrupt the cycle of compulsion, and reconnect with your body in ways that feel nourishing, not numbing.

This isn't about suppressing desire. It's about remembering you have a choice.

Hypoactive Sexual Desire Disorder (HSDD)

When desire goes quiet—and no one told you it had a name.

Let's talk about the most common sexual concern among women—and the one that rarely gets named out loud.

According to the Mayo Clinic, hypoactive sexual desire disorder (HSDD) is the top reason vulva-owners seek support for sexual health. But most don't even know it's a thing.

Here's what it looks like: your interest in sex has dipped—or disappeared—and it's not just a phase. You're not fantasizing. You're not

Naming What You're Feeling

initiating. You're not even feeling it when someone else tries. It's not about pain, trauma, or medication. It's just… gone. And it's messing with you.

HSDD means your sexual desire has dropped in a way that's persistent, disruptive, and distressing. It leaves you questioning yourself, your body, your relationship—or all of the above.

You might notice:

- You don't have spontaneous desire (those "I want you now" thoughts don't show up)
- You don't respond to sexual cues like you used to
- You lose interest halfway through a sexual experience
- You avoid intimacy—not out of fear, but out of flatness or disconnect
- You feel off about it all: frustrated, sad, ashamed… even grieving something you didn't know you'd miss

This condition can be lifelong, or it can sneak up on you at any point. It might show up only with certain partners or settings—or feel like a blanket "no" across the board. Either way, it's real. And it deserves care.

HSDD often travels with:

- Low self-worth
- Confidence crashes
- Relationship disconnection
- Anxiety, depression, or burnout
- Chronic conditions like diabetes, pain, or hormonal imbalance

And yes—women with HSDD tend to visit their providers more, try more prescriptions, and still walk out feeling unseen—not because their concerns aren't valid, but because the tools available don't always match the complexity of what they're going through.

But here's the shift:

Desire isn't a mystery. It's biological, psychological, emotional, and relational.

And once you understand what's been draining it, you can start to rebuild it—on your own terms.

This isn't about judgment. It's about understanding.

Not so you can perform—but so you can choose.

Thankfully, research into the neuroendocrine and psychological mechanisms behind sexual desire is catching up—offering a more holistic, embodied picture of what this condition really is... and how to meet it with compassion.

This plan will guide you back to the roots of your desire.

Not to force it—but to gently stir what may be sleeping.

With breath, movement, and presence, we'll begin the slow return to wanting—on your timeline, in your body's language.

Sexual Arousal Disorder

(Also known as Sexual Interest/Arousal Disorder)
When your body goes quiet—even when your heart's in it.

Here's the truth no one tells you:

You can love your partner, enjoy intimacy, and still feel like your sexual spark is MIA.

You're not repulsed. You're not avoiding.

You just... aren't feeling it—in your body or in your mind.

That's what sexual arousal disorder looks like.

This isn't just about low libido. It's when you consistently experience a drop (or total disappearance) in:

- Sexual thoughts or fantasies
- Interest in initiating or responding to intimacy

- Enjoyment during sexual activity
- Physical arousal—even when the context is right

For some, this shift feels like a slow fade. For others, it's like someone flipped a switch. Either way, it starts to affect how you feel about yourself, your relationship, and your sense of connection.

There are a few different ways this can show up:

- **Subjective Arousal Disorder:** Your body might be showing signs of arousal—lubrication, swelling—but you feel emotionally blank. No spark. No mental engagement. Just going through the motions.
- **Genital Arousal Disorder:** You're mentally into it—you want to feel turned on—but your body won't catch up. It's like your brain and your genitals aren't speaking. This often happens post-menopause, with things like low sensitivity or vaginal dryness.
- **Combined Arousal Disorder:** The full disconnect. No desire in the mind, no response in the body, no fire. Just empty space where there used to be spark.

And here's the key: this is only a "disorder" if it causes *you* distress.

If your current level of desire works for you—beautiful. You don't need to chase someone else's idea of "normal."

But if you feel confused, frustrated, or grieving a version of yourself that used to want more—then you deserve answers, care, and support.

This isn't about faking your way through pleasure.

It's about coming back into honest, embodied connection—with yourself, your desire, and your right to feel again.

This plan offers a place to begin.

With nervous system grounding, body-based curiosity, and gentle reconnection, you'll start to explore what arousal feels like *now*—and how to meet it on your own terms.

Sexual Aversion Disorder

When sex feels like danger—and your body says no.

This one's no longer in the official DSM lineup—but make no mistake, it's real.

Sexual Aversion Disorder (SAD) used to have its own diagnosis. Now, it's been folded into broader categories of "sexual dysfunction." Why? Because research was limited, and clinicians didn't see it often enough to give it its own diagnostic box.

But if you've experienced it, you know how real—and how intense—it can be.

SAD isn't just low desire. It's a visceral reaction to sexual contact.

We're talking fear, anxiety, disgust—even full-on panic at the thought of genital touch.

And no, that doesn't mean something is wrong with you.

It means your system has learned to treat sex as a threat.

There's still debate about how to classify it. Some therapists view it as a phobia. Others see it as a trauma response rooted in past experiences with touch, intimacy, or shame. Still others point out that neurodivergent women—especially those with ADHD or Autism—may experience heightened sensory sensitivity, making sexual experiences feel overwhelming or distressing.

The cause may differ, but the impact is real.

And it deserves more than a label. It deserves compassion.

There are two primary ways this tends to show up:

- **Lifelong Aversion:** You've never felt good about sex. Maybe you were raised in a shame-heavy environment. Maybe you absorbed the message that sex was "dirty," "wrong," or "just for men." There may be no single traumatic event—just a lifetime of not feeling safe or curious in your sexuality.
- **Acquired Aversion:** Things were fine... until they weren't. Something shifted—trauma, rejection, a toxic dynamic—and now your body recoils. You might avoid sex altogether. You might feel nauseous at the idea of being touched. You might be fine in some contexts, but shut down in others.

What matters isn't the category—it's the lived experience.

If sex triggers dread instead of desire, that's not just "in your head." It's your body protecting you—or your brain responding to overwhelm.

This isn't about being dramatic. It's not about being "too sensitive."

It's about the brilliant, adaptive ways your nervous system has learned to keep you safe.

And yes—healing is possible.

But first, it needs a name. Then it needs gentleness.

This plan offers you a way back—slow, steady, and safe.

Not to push past fear, but to build new pathways to safety, presence, and maybe one day, pleasure. On your terms.

Sexual Pain is Real.

Before we talk about penetration, let's talk about truth.

First things first: sexual pain is real. Very real.

If you've ever been dismissed, minimized, or told it's "just in your head," please hear me now:

I believe you. I will not gaslight you.

Painful sex is not imagined. It is not a personal failure.

It is your body speaking—and it deserves to be heard.

While the somatic and nervous system practices in this book have helped many women reduce pain and rediscover pleasure, they are not a one-size-fits-all fix. Sexual pain can have many roots.

Sometimes, pain stems from being under-aroused before penetration. Sometimes, it's about not having enough lubrication. And no—being "wet" isn't the gold standard of readiness. Lube is your friend. Use it generously. Use it often. For penetration, for vulva touch, for anything involving friction. A high-quality silicone-based lubricant can make a world of difference—and it's not just for "sensitive" moments. It's for every moment where your body deserves ease.

Arousal takes time. It's not a switch—it's a sequence.

And if you're skipping ahead, your body might be throwing on the brakes for a reason.

But that's only part of the picture. Many vulva-owners experiencing sexual pain are living with undiagnosed medical conditions, such as endometriosis, pelvic floor dysfunction, or spinal cord issues. And if that pain persists, it's not because you're not "trying hard enough." It's because your body may be asking for more support.

So, as you move through this book—building in more time, more lubrication, more clitoral stimulation, and more embodied care—I also strongly encourage you to seek a medical evaluation from a provider who specializes in sexual health if your pain continues.

Your pleasure matters. So does your pain.

Both deserve to be met with understanding.

If you've already seen a primary care provider or gynecologist and left feeling unheard—or worse, dismissed—you are not alone. Many providers care deeply, but may not have the training or time to explore complex sexual health issues. That's why I recommend seeking care from a sexual health physician trained to look deeper. You can search for providers through the International Society for the Study of Women's Sexual Health (ISSWSH). Or connect with Dr. Irwin Goldstein's team at San Diego Sexual Medicine, where free consultations are available.

You can find direct links to these resources in the Trusted Clinical Resources section at the end of the book—no need to go searching.

You are not broken. You are not imagining things.

You deserve care that honors your body, your story, and your truth.

Now that we've named what's real, let's look more closely at the many ways sexual pain can speak through the body—and what it might be trying to say.

The Penetrative Disorders

When entering the body brings pain instead of pleasure.

Let's talk about pain—and not the kind you can shake off.

These conditions aren't about not being "in the mood."

They're about real, physical discomfort that shows up *every time* something tries to enter your body—whether it's a penis, a toy, a finger, a tampon, or even a speculum at the doctor's office.

And it's not just physical. It reaches into your emotions, your relationships, and your willingness to even try again.

And for many, that avoidance comes with grief, confusion, or shame—feelings no one talks about, but that register somatically, held deep in the body.

This isn't in your head.

These conditions are common, often misunderstood, and very, very real.

Dyspareunia

When penetration brings pain—and no one can tell you why.

Dyspareunia is the clinical term for persistent or recurring pain during sexual penetration—whether at the vaginal opening, deeper in the vaginal canal, around the cervix, or in the pelvis.

This pain might show up at the entrance, deeper inside, or both.

It's not vaginismus. It's not just "dryness."

And it's not because you're doing it wrong.

Often, even physical exams don't reveal a clear cause. But your body knows something's off. And that knowing deserves to be trusted.

What it might look like:

- Ongoing pain during intercourse or any penetration
- Discomfort at the vaginal opening or deep in the pelvis
- Normal medical tests, but the pain persists
- Emotional distress, disconnection, or relationship tension as a result of the pain

And if it hurts—but you keep going through with it anyway, out of guilt, pressure, or fear of rejection—your body will keep shutting down.

This is not your body betraying you.

This is your body protecting you.

It's a signal to pause, not push through.

This plan will guide you in reconnecting with safety, sensation, and self-trust—so you can begin listening to your body instead of overriding it. Pleasure is still possible. But only when pain is honored first.

Vaginismus

When your body says no—and you don't know why.

This isn't "in your head." It's in your muscles—and they're not cooperating.

Vaginismus occurs when the pelvic floor muscles reflexively and involuntarily clamp up anytime something tries to enter the vagina. This isn't a conscious choice. You're not "too uptight." You're experiencing a nervous system response your body learned somewhere along the way—often through trauma, fear, shame, or simply never being taught how to feel safe in your own body.

What it can feel like:

- A sharp, well-defined pain right at the vaginal entrance
- Your body tensing, tightening, or outright resisting anything inserted
- Trouble with tampons, fingers, sex toys, or penetrative sex
- A spasm that feels automatic—and not something you can just "breathe through"

This can happen whether you're calm or anxious. It can appear suddenly or be there from the beginning. But if penetration feels more like a wall than a doorway, this may be what you're dealing with.

The good news? Your body isn't broken.

It's responding exactly as it was trained to.

And with gentleness, time, and nervous system retraining, it can learn a new way.

This plan is about reconnecting—not forcing.

You'll begin with safety, stay with sensation, and slowly build trust in your body again, one breath at a time.

Vulvodynia

When the pain is real—but the tests say otherwise.

When pain lingers in places it shouldn't—and refuses to give you answers—that's vulvodynia.

This isn't about "sensitivity." It's about chronic, burning, stinging, maddening pain around the vulva—especially near the vaginal opening—that often comes without a clear diagnosis. It might show up out of nowhere, or be triggered by something as simple as tight jeans, underwear seams, a bike seat, or even sitting too long.

You might be dealing with vulvodynia if:

- You feel burning, rawness, or stinging in the vulva
- Pain is provoked by pressure—like from tampons, sex, clothing, or movement
- Medical tests come back "normal," but the pain is very real
- You've tried treatments that didn't help—or left you feeling dismissed

This condition is often misunderstood—not just by those experiencing it, but by the professionals trying to treat it. When nothing shows up on labs or scans, many providers are left without a clear path forward. That doesn't mean they don't care—it means the tools they've been given may not be enough. But if you've ever walked away from an appointment feeling dismissed or disheartened, please know this: you're not imagining things. Vulvodynia is real, and it deserves compassionate, informed care.

This condition can feel isolating, invisible, and relentless. But you're not imagining it—and you're not alone.

This plan won't offer a miracle cure. But it will help you come back to your body with gentleness, build nervous system resilience, and begin unwinding the pain pattern—one layer at a time, with no pressure to push past what hurts.

Vaginal Atrophy

(Also known as Genitourinary Syndrome of Menopause)
When hormones shift, and so does your body's readiness for touch.

Estrogen plays a big role in vaginal health—and when levels drop, especially after menopause, your tissues start to change. The walls of the vagina can become thinner, drier, and more fragile. That's vaginal atrophy. And it can make penetration feel like sandpaper on skin.

What it often looks like:

- Vaginal dryness or irritation—even outside of sex
- A feeling of friction, tightness, or burning with insertion
- Pain at the vaginal opening—sometimes even with lubrication
- Less elasticity or stretch in the vaginal walls

You're not imagining this.

It's a physical, hormone-driven shift—not a personal failing.

And while it's common, that doesn't mean you just have to "deal with it."

This plan will guide you through body-based tools that support tissue health, blood flow, and arousal—while also encouraging you to seek support from a menopause-informed provider if hormone therapy might be helpful for you.

Relief is possible. So is pleasure. Let's start where you are.

Your Body Is Changing—And You Still Deserve Pleasure

If you're in perimenopause or menopause, hormone changes may be part of the picture. Low estrogen, testosterone, or progesterone levels can directly impact desire, arousal, lubrication, and orgasm. These shifts can also make penetration painful.

If you suspect hormones may be playing a role in your experience, I encourage you to consult a certified menopause specialist. There are FDA-approved and off-label options available to treat the sexual symptoms of menopause—including vaginal dryness, tissue changes, and shifts in desire. These medications are well-studied and, for many women, highly effective.

That's not the same as being handed an antidepressant because you've lost interest in sex. While SSRIs and other medications can be incredibly helpful when prescribed thoughtfully, they're not a blanket fix for desire. A provider trained in sexual medicine or menopause care will consider your full picture—your hormones, your stress, your symptoms, and your satisfaction.

I'm not against pharmaceuticals. I advocate for thoughtful, individualized care—especially when it comes to your pleasure, or the lack thereof.

You can find qualified professionals through The North American Menopause Society (NAMS) and filter by location and specialty. You'll find the direct link in the Trusted Clinical Resources section at the back of this book.

Endometriosis/Pelvic Adhesions

When the pain is deep—and doesn't show up on the surface.
This is the pain you can't quite reach—and that most people don't understand.

Endometriosis and pelvic adhesions can cause internal pain that feels sharp, shocking, or like something's being "bumped" deep inside you. This isn't surface-level discomfort. It's pelvic pain that hits hard—especially with deeper penetration—and can leave you bracing for impact.

What's happening?

Tissue that should stay inside the uterus starts to grow where it doesn't belong—on the ovaries, fallopian tubes, bladder, or bowel. In some cases, past infections or surgeries leave behind scar tissue that creates similar pain patterns.

Naming What You're Feeling

You might be dealing with this if:

- You feel deep, aching, or stabbing pain during or after penetration
- The pain feels like something is hitting or bumping the wrong spot
- It intensifies with your cycle—especially around menstruation
- You don't feel burning or itchiness—this is deep, not surface-level
- You experience spotting after penetration

This condition is often missed or misunderstood—not because no one cares, but because it's hard to detect without specialized testing. And too many women have been trained to tolerate pain during their period or during sex without question.

But this kind of pain isn't normal. It's not in your head. And it sure as hell isn't something to "relax through."

This is structural. Internal. Medical.

And until the body is properly supported and heard, pleasure may remain out of reach.

This plan won't treat endo or adhesions directly—but it *will* help you reconnect with your pelvic bowl, soften protective tension, and reclaim agency over how you relate to sensation. That, too, is a kind of healing.

And if you haven't already, I encourage you to explore care from a provider who specializes in pelvic pain. Surgical treatment for endometriosis and pelvic floor physical therapy can be life-changing when this kind of pain is present. You deserve care that sees the whole picture—*and* offers real support.

Where We Go from Here

These challenges may be common—but that doesn't make them simple. And it certainly doesn't make them your fault. Each of the conditions you've just explored represents a real experience with a real impact—and now, you have a clearer understanding of what's been happening in your body. That's powerful.

But we're not stopping at insight. We're moving toward healing.

Next, we'll turn to the quieter barriers—the emotional, relational, and psychological layers that can shape everything from desire to trust to self-worth.

Chapter 13

The Quiet Barriers to Pleasure

When everything "should" be working—but something still feels off.

We've covered the physical side—the pain, the tension, the diagnoses that can make penetration uncomfortable or impossible.

But for many women, the real issue isn't just pain.

It's disconnection.

It's that foggy, shut-down feeling. The sense of being numb, checked out, emotionally distant from your own body—even when everything looks fine on paper.

Here's the truth: you don't need a medical diagnosis to be struggling.

You can still feel stuck, flat, frustrated, or unreachable.

You can still carry invisible blocks that make pleasure feel miles away.

Stress. Shame. Body image. Trauma. Conditioning.

They all live in the body. And they all shape how we experience sex.

This chapter goes beyond symptoms.

We're stepping into the quiet places—the stories beneath the skin, the nervous system imprints, the emotional echoes that never quite got resolved.

Because the path to pleasure isn't just physical.

It's emotional. It's relational. It's deeply personal.

And once you begin to name what's been standing in the way, you can start making space for something more true. More alive. More *you*.

Sexual Pleasure Barriers

What's getting in the way of feeling good?

We all want to feel good in our bodies—and in our relationships. But for many women, emotional and psychological blocks quietly take up the space where pleasure is meant to live.

Sometimes these barriers are loud and obvious.

Sometimes they're buried under years of stress, shame, or survival mode.

Either way, they're real. And they matter.

The chart below offers a snapshot of common pleasure blockers—and how they might sound or feel in everyday life. As you read through, see if any of these ring true.

Which One Do You See in Yourself?

Barrier	What It Might Feel Like
Low Self-Esteem	"I'm not enough." "They'll leave if they really know me."
Poor Body Image	"I hate how I look." "I avoid mirrors or being seen naked."

Self-Love Struggles	"I take care of everyone else but don't know how to care for myself."
Unrecognized Trauma	"I pull away when things get too close." "I get edgy for no reason."

Think of this as a mirror, not a diagnosis.

There's no pressure to label yourself—just an invitation to notice what's true for you.

Where's the Disconnect?

Sometimes, what looks like a "sex problem" isn't about sex at all.

It's about disconnection—that invisible gap between what you want to feel and what your body can actually access.

Here's what that disconnect might look like:

- Your thoughts are full of self-doubt, criticism, or shame
- Your emotions are shut down—or overwhelmed with anxiety
- Your body is numb, tense, or unresponsive—even when you want to feel more

This isn't about blame.

It's about *awareness with compassion.*

Because once you can name what's happening inside you—without judgment—you give yourself the power to shift it.

You begin to rebuild the bridge between mind, body, and heart. And that's when healing—and pleasure—can finally start to flow.

Sometimes, it helps to see it mapped out.

Here's how the disconnect might show up across your inner landscape:

Awaken Your Body Awaken Your Desire

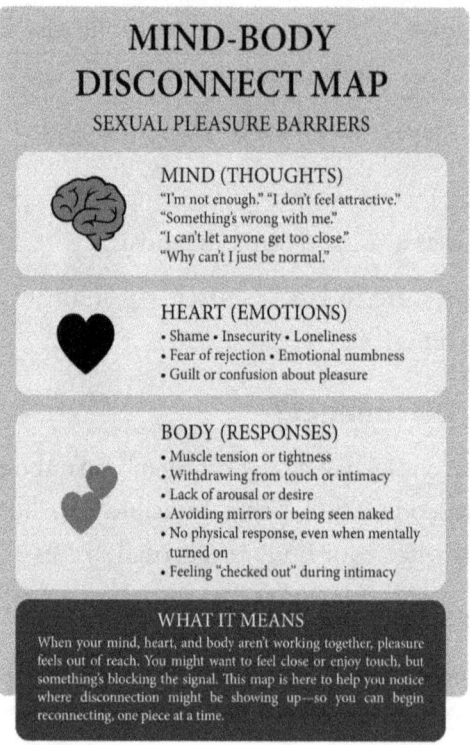

Let's Go Deeper

The barriers you've seen so far aren't abstract—they live in your thoughts, habits, and the way you move through your relationships.

They shape how you see yourself.

How safe you feel in your own skin.

How open you are to being seen, held, touched.

The pages that follow will take you more deeply into each one. You might recognize pieces of yourself in more than one category—and that's okay. These aren't boxes to fit into.

They're doorways to understanding.

Low Self Esteem

When you doubt your worth, desire has nowhere to land.

The Quiet Barriers to Pleasure

When you don't feel good about yourself, it's hard to fully show up in intimacy. Low self-esteem can quietly affect everything from how you respond to touch… to whether you even feel worthy of it.

It might look like:

- Feeling like you're not "enough" or that you don't measure up
- Struggling with self-worth, or feeling undeserving of pleasure
- Constant self-doubt, impostor syndrome—or its flip side: feeling like others can't live up to your standards (as a form of protection)
- Avoiding vulnerability or closeness because deep down, you don't believe you'll be accepted

This isn't a character flaw. It's often a response to years of messaging that taught you to question your enoughness.

But those messages can be rewritten.

And your body can learn a new truth.

Poor Body Image

When your own reflection feels like the enemy.

It's hard to feel sexy when you're at war with your own body.

Body image struggles can make intimacy feel like exposure—something to brace for, not something to enjoy.

This can show up as:

- Constantly comparing yourself to impossible standards—or heavily edited images online
- Feeling uncomfortable with your size, shape, or features, even when others reassure you
- Obsessing over things you can't change (like hair texture, skin tone, or body type) and believing they make you "less than"
- Criticizing yourself for features that are entirely natural—or deeply cultural

When you feel like your body isn't "enough," it's easy to disconnect from sensation.

To armor up.

To shrink instead of soften.

But you were never the problem.

The lens was.

And that lens can be lovingly, slowly changed.

Self-Love

When you give to everyone else—but feel starved inside.

Even when we're surrounded by people who care, it's possible to feel empty.

Anxious.

Like you're always chasing love or approval but never quite receiving it.

Self-love struggles can quietly drain your capacity for intimacy. Because when you don't feel worthy of tenderness, it's hard to let it in.

It might look like:

- Craving constant reassurance, even when love is present
- Feeling undeserving of affection, attention, or rest
- Taking care of everyone else while your own needs go unmet
- Struggling with people-pleasing, perfectionism, or anxious attachment

This isn't neediness or dysfunction—it's a nervous system shaped by survival.

You learned to stay connected by overextending yourself.

But you're allowed to unlearn that now.

You're allowed to belong to yourself first.

The Quiet Barriers to Pleasure

Unrecognized Trauma

When something in you flinches—and you're not sure why.

Sometimes, past experiences stay hidden—but they still shape how we show up in the present.

Even if the trauma hasn't been processed, named, or even consciously remembered, it can leave deep imprints on the body and nervous system.

These wounds go by many names:

Unprocessed trauma. Unspoken trauma. Invisible trauma.

Whatever the label, the impact is real.

You might notice:

- Pulling away from loved ones—especially when things get intimate or emotionally charged
- Feeling edgy, easily startled, or hyper-aware of your environment
- Trouble sleeping, unsettling dreams, or mood swings that seem to come out of nowhere
- A deep sense that your body, or your relationships, just aren't safe

This is not weakness. It's your body doing exactly what it was wired to do: protect you.

But protection doesn't have to mean disconnection.

There are gentler ways to feel safe again—ways that honor your pace, your story, and your agency.

Note for Practitioners:

This section invites attunement, not urgency.

Disclosure may unfold—but only when safety is felt, not forced.

Trust is built in the small moments. Move with reverence. Let the pace belong to the client.

Coming Back to Yourself

You've just walked through some of the most tender terrain in this book—not the obvious wounds, but the quiet ones. The ones that live beneath your skin, in your self-perception, your nervous system, your story.

Maybe you saw yourself in one section.

Maybe in all of them.

Maybe you're still unpacking what landed.

That's okay.

This isn't about rushing to fix yourself.

It's about seeing what's been hidden—and holding it with care.

Now, it's time to gather the pieces.

Everything you've uncovered—your stress, your desire, your pain, your pleasure—it all belongs. It's all part of the same story. Your story.

And what comes next?

Not a return to the person you were before—

but a movement toward the version of you who feels safe, soft, and fully alive in their body.

A Note on Clinical & Diagnostic Integrity

While this book takes a warm, plain-language approach to discussing sexual health, the terms used throughout Chapters 12 and 13 reflect both medical and psychological concerns, as defined by leading frameworks in sexual medicine and mental health. Wherever possible, I've translated these terms into accessible language—without losing the clinical meaning behind them.

These descriptions are informed by evidence-based research, current diagnostic criteria, and the lived experiences of those navigating desire, pain, disconnection, and trauma. I've also integrated insights from trauma-informed pelvic therapy and mind-body approaches to honor the multifaceted nature of women's sexual wellness.

These chapters are not intended to replace a medical or psychological evaluation. They're here to offer clarity, compassion, and a more complete understanding of your experience—so you can move forward with greater insight and agency.

If you're looking for additional support, you'll find vetted referrals and guidance in the *Trusted Clinical Resources* section at the end of the book.

Let's keep going. You're ready.

PART 3
YOUR HEALING PLAN

Chapter 14

The Somatic Toolkit

Breath, Movement, and Meditation for Reclaiming Your Body

This chapter gathers all the body-based practices we've introduced throughout the book—fully detailed, clearly laid out, and ready for you to use. Think of it as your personal somatic toolkit: a resource to support embodiment, regulation, and reconnection.

These pages aren't meant to be read in a single sitting—they're here to be explored, returned to, and woven into your healing rhythm over time.

Inside this chapter, you'll find:

- Breathwork techniques to calm, energize, or rebalance your nervous system
- Yoga postures that awaken sensation and build strength, openness, and body awareness
- Meditation practices that anchor you in presence and internal safety

Glance through all the options now, just to get a feel for what's here. Then, once you've read your personalized Healing Plan(s) in Chapter 16, come back and study your recommended breathwork, postures, and meditation practices. Return as often as you need—whether to revisit your assigned tools or to explore new ones as your body calls for more.

You won't need to use everything at once. But over time, you may find yourself drawn to expand your practice. Let this chapter grow with you—offering more when you're ready.

This section is designed to be used alongside your Healing Plan, again and again, as your needs shift and your relationship to your body deepens.

If you're reading the digital version, you might want to print some pages for off-screen guidance. If you're using a physical copy, consider bookmarking this section so it's easy to return to when you practice.

This is your body's reference guide.

Come back whenever you need to breathe, move, or soften back into yourself.

The Breathwork Techniques

Your breath is more than just air—it's information.

It tells your nervous system whether you're safe or threatened, relaxed or bracing for impact. And when you use it intentionally, it becomes one of the most powerful healing tools you have.

Breathe Like You Mean It

Let's start with breath.

You can't overanalyze your way into desire—but you can breathe your way into it.

Before you try to "fix" your sex life, there's one thing you need to understand: your breath is your baseline.

It's the first thing to slip away when you're stressed, shut down, or disconnected from your body. And it's the first thing you can control to bring yourself back home.

You'll find 13 powerful breathwork techniques in this section (one appears twice—for good reason), each carefully matched to a specific sexual health concern or emotional barrier. This isn't woo-woo nonsense—and it's definitely not generic self-care fluff.

There are hundreds of breathing exercises out there, but I've curated the ones that most directly support your specific concern. Each one is:

- Backed by research
- Rooted in proven mind-body practices

- Matched to how your nervous system responds under stress, fear, shutdown, or overload

Whether you're dealing with low desire, trauma-related shutdown, compulsive urges, or just the pressure to "perform," your breath is one of the most direct and effective tools you've got.

For example, if you're working with vaginismus, your breathwork will look very different than someone on a healing path for hypersexuality. You don't have to figure out which one to use—I've already done that for you.

But that doesn't mean you can't try others. Your Healing Plan offers a starting point, not a limit. Feel free to explore different breathwork techniques as your body feels ready—there's no rush, just resonance.

Come back to this chapter anytime you need to reset.

The more you practice, the more your body will start to remember what it means to feel calm, safe, clear… and capable of real pleasure.

Quick Reference: Breathing Techniques by Concern

Before we dive into the step-by-step instructions, here's your cheat sheet.

As mentioned, there are 13 unique breathwork techniques in total—though Lion's Breath appears twice, because it's especially effective across more than one area of healing.

Use this table anytime you want a quick match between what you're experiencing and the breathwork that best supports it.

Concern/Barrier	Breathing Technique
1. Hypoactive Sexual Desire (HSDD)	Breath of Fire
2. Sexual Arousal Disorder	Lion's Breath
3. Sexual Aversion Disorder	Box Breathing

The Breathwork Techniques

Concern/Barrier	Breathing Technique
4. Hypersexuality (HCSB)	Alternate Nostril Breathing
5. Anorgasmia	Breath of Joy
6. Dyspareunia (DYS)	Abdominal Breathing
7. Vaginismus (VAG)	Cooling Breath
8. Vulvodynia	Bee Breath
9. Endometriosis	4-7-8 Breathing
10. Vaginal Atrophy (VA)	Three-Part Breath
11. Low Self-Esteem (LSE)	Bellows Breath
12. Poor Body Image (PBI)	Equal Breathing
13. Unrecognized Trauma (UT)	Ocean Breath
14. Self-Love	Lion's Breath

You'll find the full breakdown of each technique in the pages that follow.

1. Breath of Fire *(for HSDD – low sexual desire)*

A rapid, rhythmic breath through the nose that builds energy and awakens the body.

- Stimulates circulation
- Builds internal heat
- Sparks motivation and desire

2. Lion's Breath *(for arousal challenges & self-love barriers)*

A powerful exhale with the tongue out and a loud "ha" sound.

- Releases inner pressure
- Boosts confidence and expression
- Helps you reclaim boldness

3. Box Breathing *(for Sexual Aversion Disorder)*
Inhale, hold, exhale, hold—each for an equal count.

- Calms anxiety
- Creates safety and structure
- Helps regain emotional control

4. Alternate Nostril Breathing *(for compulsive sexual urges)*
A balancing breath that shifts energy between the two sides of the brain.

- Reduces overstimulation
- Supports self-regulation
- Helps quiet obsessive thoughts

5. Breath of Joy *(for Anorgasmia)*
Three quick inhales and one strong exhale with movement.

- Lifts low mood
- Shakes off emotional heaviness
- Reinvites joy and pleasure

6. Abdominal Breathing *(for Dyspareunia)*
A slow, deep breath focused on expanding the belly.

- Relaxes pelvic floor tension
- Reduces pain signals
- Encourages body trust

7. Cooling Breath *(for Vaginismus)*
Inhale through a curled tongue or pursed lips; exhale slowly.

- Lowers internal heat and stress
- Soothes sensitivity
- Softens hyper-alert muscle tension

8. Bee Breath *(for Vulvodynia)*
A slow, deep inhale followed by a long humming exhale.

- Vibrations calm the brain
- Eases nervous tension
- Supports sensory reset

9. 4-7-8 Breathing *(for Endometriosis)*
Inhale for 4, hold for 7, exhale for 8.

- Calms the entire system
- Helps manage pain and tension
- Supports rest, sleep, and hormonal regulation

10. Three-Part Breath *(for Vaginal Atrophy)*
Breathing into the belly, ribs, and chest—one layer at a time.

- Brings awareness to underused areas
- Gently expands inner tissue
- Improves oxygen flow to the pelvic region

11. Bellows Breath *(for Low Self-Esteem)*
Fast, sharp breaths through the nose to build internal fire.

- Increases energy
- Boosts confidence
- Helps push through emotional heaviness

12. Equal Breathing *(for Poor Body Image)*
Match your inhale and exhale lengths, keeping them slow and steady.

- Creates balance
- Anchors you in the present
- Promotes body neutrality and calm

13. Ocean Breath (Ujjayi) *(for Unrecognized Trauma)*
A soft, constricted breath that sounds like waves in the back of your throat.

- Regulates trauma responses

- Grounds awareness in the body
- Brings calm to a dysregulated nervous system

Each breath has its own rhythm.

Pick the one that matches your current need—or the one your body quietly says yes to.

Next up: we'll break down how to do each of these breathwork techniques, step by step.

Use this chapter like a personal guidebook—come back whenever you need a reset.

The Breathwork Techniques

1. Breath of Fire

Sanskrit: Kapalabhati Pranayama *(Kapālabhāti Prāṇāyāma)*

Best For: Hypoactive Sexual Desire Disorder (HSDD)

Breath of Fire is bold, bright, and unapologetically activating. This isn't a sleepy inhale-exhale meditation—it's a powerful, rhythmic breath that clears your head, stokes your inner fire, and wakes up the body from the inside out.

It strengthens the core, activates the sexual muscles, and gets blood flowing to the areas that need it most. It's a breath for stirring desire—on every level.

How to Practice:

1. Sit tall in a comfortable position—cross-legged is great, but any upright seat will do.
2. Rest your hands on your knees, palms up. Want to feel the movement? Place one hand on your belly if that feels good.
3. Inhale deeply through your nose. Let your belly expand.
4. Without pausing, exhale sharply through your nose while snapping your belly in (like you're firing the air out).
5. Let the inhales happen passively, and focus on the sharp, active exhale.
6. Once you've got the rhythm, speed it up—short, equal bursts in and out through the nose.
7. Do this for 30 seconds to start. Gradually increase your time as your stamina builds—but don't exceed 5 minutes in one session.

A Note on Safety:

This breath is intense. Skip it if you're pregnant, have uncontrolled hypertension, or are recovering from recent abdominal surgery. Listen to your body. Always.

2. Lion's Breath

Sanskrit: Simha Pranayama *(Siṁha Prāṇāyāma)*

Best For: Sexual Arousal Disorder and Self-Love Challenges

Lion's Breath is bold, expressive, and unapologetically alive. It's a breath that invites you to shake off tension, awaken your senses, and reclaim space—in your body and your heart.

If you're struggling with arousal, this practice helps jumpstart physical energy and emotional presence. If you're navigating self-love wounds, it creates space to roar out shame and reconnect with your confidence. Either way, it helps you come home to yourself with fire and freedom.

How to Practice:

1. Sit in a strong, stable position—cross-legged, kneeling, or seated in a chair. Feel grounded.
2. Lean forward slightly, placing your hands on your knees or thighs. Spread your fingers wide—like claws.
3. Inhale deeply through your nose, filling your belly and chest.
4. Open your mouth wide. Stick your tongue out and down toward your chin.
5. Exhale with a powerful "haaaa" sound, pulling the breath from your belly. Let the sound be fierce.
6. Pause and breathe normally for a few moments.
7. Repeat Lion's Breath 5–7 times, or until you feel something shift.
8. After your final round, sit in stillness and breathe deeply for 1–3 minutes to integrate.

Pro Tip: Let this breath be messy and real. Shake your head, wag your metaphorical tail, or roar softly if it helps. This is your moment to clear space—emotionally, physically, and energetically.

Whether you're reigniting desire or reclaiming your worth, Lion's Breath is here to remind you that you are allowed to take up space—loudly, fully, and without apology.

3. Box Breathing

Sanskrit: Sama Vritti Pranayama *(Samavṛtti Prāṇāyāma)*

Best For: Sexual Aversion Disorder

When anxiety hijacks your body or your thoughts, Box Breathing brings you back into control. This practice uses a steady, four-part breath to quiet the mind, settle the nervous system, and help you feel safe in your own skin again.

Box Breathing is widely used by clinicians, first responders, and athletes for one reason: it works. It's especially powerful for those who've experienced trauma or feel a heightened startle response around intimacy or touch.

How to Practice:

1. Find a comfortable seat. Sit tall but relaxed. Let your hands rest softly.
2. Exhale fully through your mouth, releasing all the air in your lungs.
3. Inhale slowly through your nose for a count of 4. Let the breath fill your belly, ribs, and chest.
4. Hold the breath for a count of 4.
5. Exhale slowly through your mouth for a count of 4.
6. Hold again for 4.
7. Repeat the cycle 4–6 times, or for up to 5 minutes.

Extra Tip:

Visualize a box as you breathe—inhale up one side, hold across the top, exhale down the other side, hold across the bottom. Let each corner ground you in calm, intentional awareness.

4. Alternate Nostril Breathing

Sanskrit: Nadi Shodhana Pranayama *(Nāḍī Śodhana Prāṇāyāma)*

Best For: Hypersexuality / Compulsive Sexual Behavior

When your mind is racing, your body's overstimulated, or you feel stuck in an all-or-nothing pattern—this breath will bring you back to center.

Alternate Nostril Breathing is one of the most effective ways to reset your nervous system. It balances the left and right hemispheres of the brain, regulates energy flow, and creates a natural rhythm that clears mental chaos and soothes the body.

How to Practice:

1. Sit comfortably, either cross-legged or in a chair with both feet on the ground. Keep your spine long and your shoulders relaxed.
2. Place your left hand on your left knee. Bring your right hand up to your face.
3. Close your right nostril with your right thumb.
4. Inhale slowly through your left nostril.
5. Close your left nostril with your ring finger.
6. Open your right nostril and exhale fully through the right side.
7. Inhale through your right nostril.
8. Close your right nostril, then open the left and exhale.

That's one full cycle. Continue for 3–5 minutes, finishing with an exhale on the left side.

Important Note:

This is not a race. Go slow. Focus on smooth transitions and steady breath. The goal is balance—not sedation, not stimulation—just steady presence.

5. Breath of Joy

Sanskrit: None—modern breath-movement practice

Best For: Anorgasmia

Sometimes, the quickest way to shift your state is to move your body and breathe like you mean it. Breath of Joy does both. This dynamic practice opens your chest, lifts your energy, and clears out emotional heaviness. It's especially powerful when you're feeling flat, stuck, or disconnected from pleasure.

You can practice Breath of Joy standing or seated—what matters most is that you move with intention and exhale with gusto.

How to Practice

Setup (Standing or Seated):

- Stand with your feet shoulder-width apart, knees slightly bent, and chest open.
- Or sit tall in a sturdy chair, feet grounded, with enough room to move your arms freely.

Movement + Breath Sequence:

1. Inhale 1/3 of your lung capacity as you swing your arms forward—palms facing up, shoulder height.
2. Inhale 2/3 as you sweep your arms out wide to the sides—like wings, still shoulder height.
3. Inhale to full capacity as you swing your arms overhead—palms facing each other.
4. Exhale loudly through your mouth ("ha!") as you swing your arms down and back behind you.
   - If standing, bend your knees deeply like you're diving.
   - If seated, hinge forward from your hips, letting your arms sweep behind you.

The Breathwork Techniques

Repeat 7–9 times, letting the movement and breath sync up naturally.

Tips for Practice:
- Try the motions a few times without breath first, just to get the rhythm.
- Then bring in the breath—and the joy.
- Don't force or strain. This is about freedom, fluidity, and letting go.

Let yourself play. Let yourself breathe. Let yourself feel the energy move through you.

Note: If you feel lightheaded, pause and return to normal breathing. Start slowly and increase repetitions over time.

6. Abdominal Breathing

Sanskrit: Adham Pranayama *(Adhama Prāṇāyāma)*

Best For: Dyspareunia

Also known as belly breathing or diaphragmatic breathing, this technique teaches your body how to expand, soften, and let go. It's simple but powerful—especially when pain, fear, or tension are lingering in the pelvic floor.

Abdominal breathing has been shown to lower cortisol levels (your primary stress hormone), which directly impacts how the body perceives pain. When you breathe deeply into your belly, you're not just calming your mind—you're rewiring your nervous system's response to discomfort.

How to Practice:

1. Sit or lie down on a flat, comfortable surface. Grab a blanket if you run cold. Settle in.
2. Relax your shoulders—gently draw them away from your ears.
3. Place your right hand on your chest and your left hand on your abdomen.
4. Inhale deeply through your nose without straining, filling your lungs as much as possible.
5. Feel your abdomen rise and expand, while your chest remains mostly still.
6. Purse your lips like you're sipping through a straw. Exhale slowly for a count of 4, letting your belly release gently toward your spine.
7. Repeat for 10–50 breath cycles, or as long as feels good.

Use This Practice When:

- You're feeling overwhelmed or emotionally tense
- You're preparing for intimacy or navigating pain

- You want to gently reconnect with your body and feel grounded

This is the breath that brings you home. Gentle, steady, and deeply supportive—let it become your go-to during any moment of distress, or as a daily ritual for nervous system regulation.

7. Cooling Breath

Sanskrit: Sheetali Pranayama *(Śītali Prāṇāyāma)*

Best For: Vaginismus

As the name suggests, Cooling Breath is designed to bring a gentle wave of calm through your system. It soothes heat, irritation, and tension—not just physically, but emotionally. It's especially helpful when your body is in a high-sensitivity state and pressure (internal or external) makes relaxation feel impossible.

Practiced regularly, Śītalī trains your nervous system to downshift and teaches your muscles how to release. And when your body learns to unwind? Your mind often follows.

How to Practice:

1. Sit in a stable, supported position. Cross-legged or in a chair—whatever helps you feel at ease.
2. Relax your shoulders and close your eyes if comfortable. Imagine a soft wave of cool air beginning to move through you.
3. Take 2–3 deep breaths in and out through your nose to settle in.
4. Stick your tongue out and roll the sides into a tube. (If you can't roll your tongue, purse your lips into a small "O" shape instead.)
5. Inhale deeply through the rolled tongue or pursed lips. Feel the cool air pass over your tongue and into your body.
6. Withdraw your tongue and exhale slowly through your nose.
7. That's one round. Repeat 8–14 times, moving slowly and steadily.

Let the soft "sipping" sensation anchor you in the moment. Let your body respond however it wants.

Use This Practice When:

- You're overheated, overstimulated, or emotionally raw
- Your pelvic floor feels tight, tense, or reactive
- You need to create a calm pause before intimacy or movement

This is a breath of softness and surrender. Let it remind you that relaxation isn't passive—it's something you can choose, build, and welcome back into your body.

8. Bee Breath

Sanskrit: Bhramari Pranayama *(Bhrāmari Prāṇāyāma)*

Best For: Vulvodynia

Bee Breath—also called Humming Bee Breath—uses sound and vibration to stimulate your vagus nerve, the superhighway of your body's calming response. When the vagus nerve is activated, your parasympathetic nervous system steps in, inviting rest, ease, and repair.

This technique creates a gentle internal hum, like a sonic massage from the inside out. It's deeply grounding, especially for those managing pain, overstimulation, or sensitivity in the pelvic region.

How to Practice:

1. Sit tall with your spine long and shoulders relaxed. Close your eyes. Let your jaw soften.
2. Bring your index fingers to the cartilage just outside your ear canal (the tragus), or gently cup your ears with your palms.
3. Inhale slowly through your nose.
4. As you exhale, make a steady, high-pitched humming sound—like a buzzing bee. Feel the vibration ripple through your skull and chest.
5. If using your fingers or palms, you can gently pulse or vary pressure on your ears to enhance the internal sound.
6. Repeat for 5 to 8 rounds. Let each hum grow softer and slower.
7. After your last exhale, rest in silence and breathe normally for 1–3 minutes.

Pro Tip: Higher-pitched hums tend to produce deeper resonance—but always stay within your comfort zone. Let the vibration be smooth, not strained.

Healing Tip: Before you shift into movement or intimacy, pause. Tune into any lingering sensation. Let the subtle vibration from the hum settle into areas of holding, like you're sending calm exactly where it's needed.

This breath doesn't ask you to force anything—it simply invites you to listen inward and soften.

9. 4-7-8 Breathing

Sanskrit: Visama Vrtti Pranayama (*Viṣama Vṛtti Prāṇāyāma*)

Best For: Endometriosis & Pelvic Adhesions

4-7-8 Breathing is a powerful technique rooted in classical *pranayama*, designed to calm the nervous system and reset the body's stress response. By extending the exhale, this method activates the parasympathetic nervous system—your body's built-in calming switch. It's particularly supportive when navigating the deep, chronic tension that endometriosis and pelvic adhesions can create.

With each breath cycle, you create more space, softness, and surrender in the body.

How to Practice:

Each round follows this rhythm:

Inhale for 4 seconds → Hold for 7 seconds → Exhale for 8 seconds

1. Sit or lie down in a comfortable, supported position.
2. Gently part your lips and exhale fully through your mouth with a soft whooshing sound.
3. Close your mouth and inhale through your nose for a count of 4.
4. Hold your breath for a count of 7.
5. Open your lips and exhale slowly through your mouth for a count of 8, making a soft whooshing sound.
6. That's one round. Begin with 4 full cycles.

Tips for Practice:

- The held breath is where your nervous system recalibrates. Allow the stillness to soften tension from the inside out.
- If the full 4-7-8 feels too long, try 2-3-4 to begin. Keep the proportions the same.

- Over time, work your way up to 8 rounds for deeper calm and better nervous system regulation.

After the Practice:

Let yourself settle in stillness. Don't rush. That quiet moment afterward is part of the medicine.

4-7-8 Breathing is known to lower cortisol, support better sleep, and reduce pain perception. Think of it as your inner reset button—one you can press anytime, anywhere.

10. Three-Part Breath

Sanskrit: Dirgha Pranayama (Dīrgha Prāṇāyāma)

Best For: Vaginal Atrophy

Three-Part Breath is a deeply nourishing technique that gently expands your breath into three distinct areas: the belly, the rib cage, and the upper chest. Each inhale creates a ripple effect through your body—a wave of breath that soothes your nervous system and reconnects you to your inner rhythm.

This practice encourages balance in your physical body, emotional mind, and spiritual grounding. For vaginal atrophy—where circulation, elasticity, and internal awareness may feel diminished—this breath reawakens your connection to your body from the inside out.

How to Practice:

You can do this lying down or seated—just choose a position that feels fully supported and safe for your body today.

1. Inhale through your nose, letting your belly rise gently as the breath fills your lower lungs.
   Exhale through your nose, lightly engaging your abdominals to draw the navel toward your spine.

2. Inhale again, this time filling your belly and your rib cage.
   Feel the sides of your body expand like wings.

   Exhale slowly, letting both the rib cage and belly empty with control.

3. Inhale once more—fill the belly, the rib cage, and then draw the breath up to your upper chest.
   Feel your collarbones lift just slightly.

   Exhale fully, releasing from the top down: chest, ribs, belly.

The Breathwork Techniques

Keep in Mind:

- Let the breath feel smooth and connected—no jerking or force.
- Visualize the breath as a wave, flowing from your pelvis up to your heart, and back down.
- Stay curious. Each round may feel different. The key is awareness, not perfection.

With regular practice, this breath can increase circulation, soften internal tension, and gently reawaken pleasure pathways.

Let it be a homecoming to your body—one breath at a time.

11. Bellows Breath

Sanskrit: Bhastrika Pranayama (Bhastrikā Prāṇāyāma)

Best For: Low Self-Esteem

Bellows Breath—also known as stimulating breath—is a powerful, energizing practice designed to awaken both your body and your spirit. It brings clarity to the mind, generates internal heat, and sparks a sense of momentum—all by activating your breath as fuel.

This technique moves energy fast. It can create a natural uplift in your mood, sharpen focus, and reconnect you with your inner strength and confidence. Over time, regular practice may help counter mental fog, emotional fatigue, and self-doubt.

How to Practice:

1. Sit comfortably in a stable, supported position—on the floor or in a chair.
2. Rest your hands on your thighs, palms facing upward.
3. Begin with a few slow, natural breaths in and out through your nose.
4. When ready, inhale deeply through your nose and pull your belly inward toward your spine.
5. Exhale forcefully through your nose while pushing your belly outward.
6. Continue this cycle:
   Inhale – belly in.

   Exhale – belly out.
7. Maintain a rhythmic pace, about one full breath per second.
8. Start with 10–20 rounds. Gradually increase as your body adapts, up to 3 rounds of 20–30 breaths.

Afterward:

Pause. Let your breathing return to normal. Notice any tingling, warmth, or movement of energy (prāṇa) through your body.

Then gently cross your arms over your chest in a self-embrace. Let that movement seal in what you've stirred—reminding yourself: You are here. You are powerful. You are enough.

12. Equal Breathing

Sanskrit: Sama Vritti Pranayama (Sama Vṛtti Prāṇāyāma)

Best For: Poor Body Image

Also known as Balanced Breathing, Sama Vritti is a deeply centering practice that brings harmony to your nervous system—and quiet to your inner critic. It's gentle, accessible, and remarkably effective at calming the mind, regulating emotions, and restoring a steady rhythm to your body.

When your thoughts are harsh or your relationship with your body feels strained, this breath helps you soften. It reminds you that you don't need to fix or force anything—you can simply come back to yourself, one even breath at a time.

How to Practice:

1. Sit in a comfortable position—cross-legged on the floor or supported in a chair. You can also lie down.
2. Gently close your eyes. Take a few natural breaths, simply noticing the pace and texture of your inhale and exhale.
3. Begin to inhale slowly to a count of 4 in your mind:
   1... 2... 3... 4.
   Pause softly at the top.
4. Exhale to the same count:
   1... 2... 3... 4.
   Pause at the bottom.
5. Repeat:
   Inhale – 1, 2, 3, 4. Pause.
   Exhale – 1, 2, 3, 4. Pause.
6. Continue this rhythmic breathing for 3–5 minutes. If comfortable, you can increase the count to 6 or 8 as your lung capacity and focus expand.

Let the breath anchor you.

Feel the steadiness, the balance, the quiet rhythm of being enough—exactly as you are.

Let this practice be a gentle reminder:

You are allowed to soften. You are safe to be in your body. You are worthy of peace.

13. Ocean Breath

Sanskrit: Ujjayi Pranayama (Ujjāyī Prāṇāyāma)

Best For: Unrecognized Trauma

Ocean Breath conjures a feeling—like waves rolling in, the scent of salt, the warmth of sunlight on your skin. Just the name invites you to slow down and return to yourself.

Also known as Ujjayi, this technique mirrors the steady rhythm of the sea and offers a grounding sensory anchor—one that calms the mind, soothes the nervous system, and invites you back into presence. It's especially supportive for those navigating trauma, anxiety, or emotional overwhelm.

With its soft, wave-like sound created at the back of the throat, Ocean Breath helps regulate your fight-or-flight response and gently reattunes your awareness back into your body.

How to Practice:

1. Sit comfortably—cross-legged, kneeling, or in a supported chair. Let your spine be tall and your body feel safe.
2. Take a few natural breaths through your nose. No need to force or change anything—just notice.
3. On your next exhale, slightly constrict the back of your throat—as if you were fogging up a mirror and close your mouth.
4. Inhale through your nose while maintaining this slight throat constriction. You should hear a soft "ocean wave" sound.
5. Continue breathing in and out through your nose, keeping that gentle closure in the throat throughout. The sound should be audible but soothing—never strained.
6. Visualize a wave drawing back as you inhale, and crashing softly to shore as you exhale.

7. Practice for 3 minutes to start. Over time, you can extend your sessions to 5–7 minutes, or use it anytime your nervous system needs a reset.

Let this be your internal shoreline.

A steady breath that pulls you back from chaos, judgment, and fragmentation—into clarity, calm, and coherence.

This is your sanctuary.

Come back to it—again and again.

The Yoga Postures

Your body is more than structure—it's a source of memory, meaning, and momentum.

Through intentional movement, you don't just stretch tissue—you shift your experience.

Each pose becomes a pathway back to sensation, safety, and self-trust.

And when practiced with presence, yoga becomes not just movement—but medicine.

Move Like You Matter

You don't have to be flexible. You don't have to be spiritual.

You just have to be willing to move like your body matters.

Because it does.

Yoga isn't just about stretching—it's about sensing.

It's a practice that brings your body, breath, and awareness into harmony. It helps you tune in, increase blood flow to the pelvic region, calm the nervous system, and release long-held muscular tension.

Yoga and meditation have been shown to increase calming brain chemicals like GABA and serotonin while lowering stress hormones like cortisol and adrenaline.

One study published in *The Journal of Sexual Medicine* found that yoga improved every domain of female sexual function— desire, arousal, lubrication, orgasm, satisfaction, and pain.

Certain postures even lengthen and strengthen the pelvic floor, reduce pain, and support more sensation during sex.

For those healing from trauma, yoga offers something rare: a structured, safe way to re-enter the body—without needing to speak.

As trauma expert Dr. Bessel van der Kolk writes, yoga helps survivors reclaim internal control and presence, allowing the body to become a place of *being*—not just protection.

When practiced regularly, the benefits of yoga don't stay on the mat. They follow you into the bedroom—bringing with them more presence, more responsiveness, and more trust in your own body.

What You'll Find in This Section

A Reference Guide to the Yoga Poses in Your Healing Plan

This section is a visual guide to every yoga pose used in the Healing Plans.

You won't find full sequences here—just individual postures, offered one at a time, so you can explore them with intention and ease.

Each pose is here to support body awareness, nervous system regulation, and embodied healing. You don't need a diagnosis to benefit from them. Every posture in this section is good for every body.

You might refer to this section when you're reviewing your Healing Plan and want to know how to do a pose.

Or you might choose a single posture and stay with it—just to see what shifts.

You can flip through until something catches your attention, or return to a favorite pose whenever your body asks for it.

Each entry includes clear instructions and simple visual guidance, reviewed by advanced yoga educators and shaped with trauma-informed care in mind.

The Yoga Postures

You'll find the postures listed alphabetically so they're easy to locate, learn from, and come back to.

There's no rush.

No right way.

Just your body, your breath, and your curiosity.

AIRPLANE POSE — Dekasana

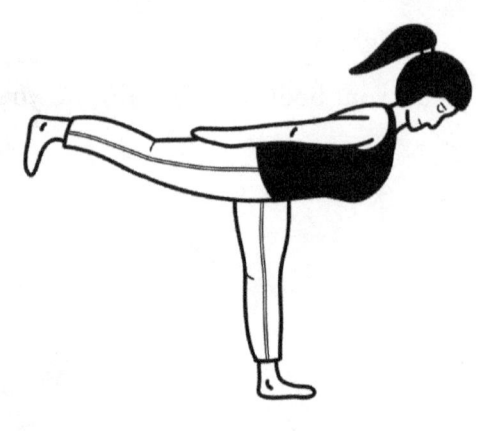

1. From Mountain Pose, Tadasana—transfer your weight into your right leg, extend your left leg back and up as you tip your torso forward.
2. Press the big toe of your supporting foot into the floor as you simultaneously lift the arch of the foot. This will help you to balance. You will also find balancing easier if you engage all the muscles of your lifted leg. Reach actively through the ball of your lifted foot.
3. Keep your hips level by rolling your left hip down and reaching the inside thigh of the left leg toward the sky.
4. Press the back of your heart forward to create an opening through your chest. You can also do this by externally rotating your arms in the shoulder sockets. Reach your arms back, extending through your fingertips, like airplane wings.
5. Gaze a few feet in front of you on the ground to help you balance and keep the back of the neck long.
6. Follow the same steps on the opposite side.
7. When you release down, stand firm in your Mountain Pose to ground yourself. Breathe.

BANANA POSE — Bananasana

1. Lie down on your back, legs straight, arms overhead.
2. With your bottom firmly anchored on the mat, move both of your legs to the right. Use your right foot to keep your left foot in place, by crossing at your ankles.
3. Bottom still anchored on the mat, bring your upper body to the right, allowing your spine to bend to the side, clasping your left wrist with your right hand. You are creating the shape of a banana with your body. Hold for 3 to 5 minutes.
4. To come out of the pose, slowly bring your body back to neutral.
5. Repeat on the opposite side.

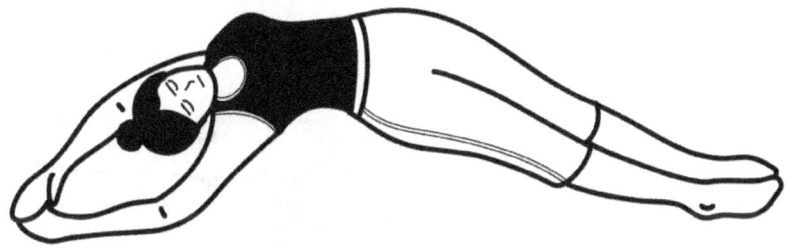

Note:

You're looking for gentle stimulation along the side body. You might feel sensations through your ribs, shoulders, or arms—and also through your hips and thighs. You may feel it in both halves of your body all at once. Send your breath to where you feel the most tension.

BIRD DOG POSE — Pārśva Bālāsana

1. Kneel on a yoga mat or blanket with your knees hip-width apart and hands firmly on the ground, about shoulder-width apart. Brace your abdominals.
2. Point one arm out straight in front and extend the opposite leg behind you, forming a straight line from your extended hand to your extended foot. Keep your hips squared to the ground. If your low back begins to sag, lower your leg until you can maintain a straight spine.
3. Hold for a few seconds, then return to your hands and knees. Keep your belly engaged throughout the entire exercise and try to minimize any extra motion in your hips during the weight shift.
4. Switch to the other side. Opposite arm, and leg.

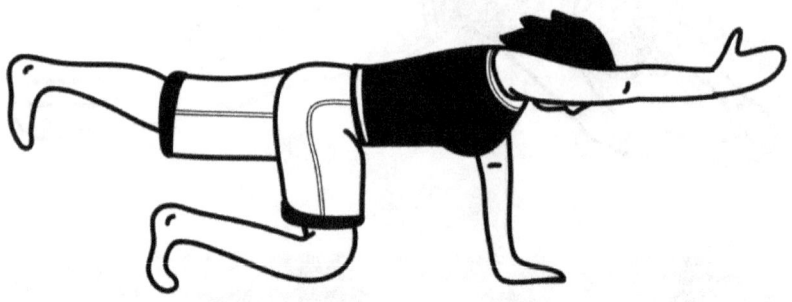

Note:

If your right arm is extended, your left leg is extended. If your left arm is extended, your right leg is extended. Always extend opposite limbs–this keeps you centered and steady.

The focus should be on forming one straight line from your hand to your foot. Your hips should be square the whole time.

CAT/COW — Marjaryasana-Bitilasana

1. Start on your hands and knees, aligning your wrists under your shoulders and your knees under your hips.
2. Think of your spine as a straight line connecting your shoulders to your hips. Visualize it extending forward through the crown of your head and back through your tailbone. This is a neutral spine.
3. Keep your neck long by looking down and out. As you inhale, arch your back into Cow Pose.

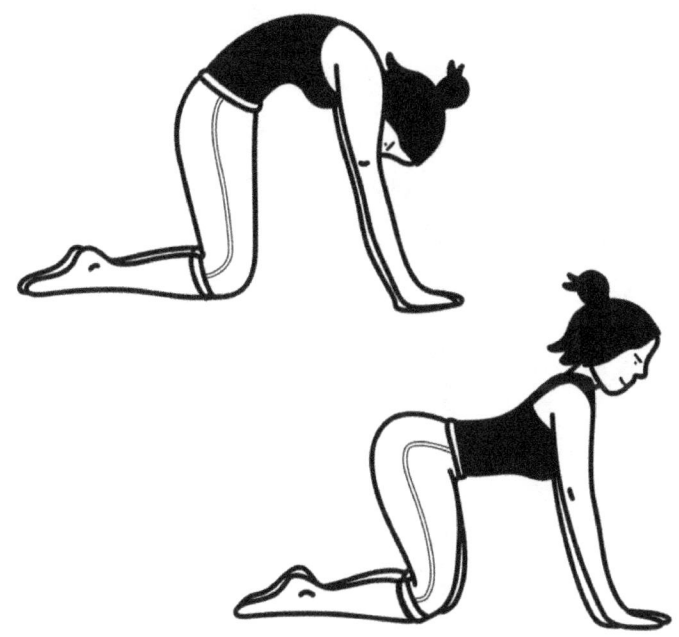

4. Curl your toes under. Tilt your pelvis back so that your tailbone lifts. Let the movement ripple up your spine, letting your neck be the last thing to move.
5. Your belly drops, but your abdominal muscles stay active – hug your spine by gently drawing your navel in.
6. Take your gaze gently upward–without cranking your neck.
7. As you exhale, round your back into Cat Pose.

8. Release the tops of your feet to the floor. Tuck your tailbone and let the movement rise up your spine. Your back will naturally round.
9. Draw your navel toward your spine. Let your head drop. Take your gaze inward–toward your navel or heart center.
10. Repeat this sequence with each inhale and exhale, moving the whole spine in rhythm with your breath. Let your breath guide the flow, sending awareness into the spine and pelvis with each cycle.
11. After your final exhale, come back to a neutral spine.

CAT/COW, SEATED
Upavistha Marjaryasana/Bitilasana

1. Sit comfortably on the floor or at the edge of a chair with your feet planted under your knees. Keep your gaze forward. Let your hands rest on your thighs or stretch your arms out to the sides.
2. As you inhale, simultaneously turn your gaze upward. Pull your belly button toward your spine and lift your chest toward the sky. If your hands are on your thighs, slide them back from your knees toward your upper thighs. This is Cow Pose.
3. As you exhale, turn your gaze down. Tuck your chin toward your chest. Round your back and pull your belly button inward. Glide your hands from your thighs back toward your knees. This is Cat Pose.
4. Continue to alternate between these two movements as you breathe in and out. Let your breath initiate the movement, and allow your spine to follow.

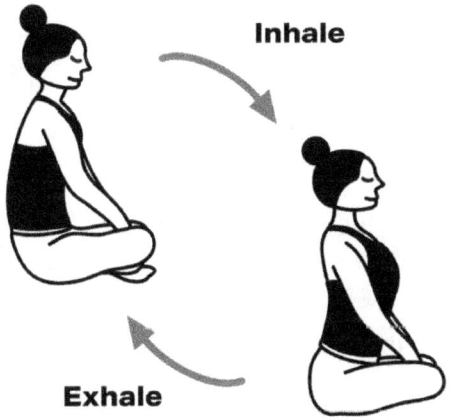

Note:
Notice the flow between expansion and contraction. Send your breath to any tight spots along your spine or neck, and feel yourself soften into the rhythm of each breath cycle.

CHAIR POSE — Utkatasana

1. Stand in Mountain Pose, (Tadasana). Inhale, raise your arms overhead so your biceps are just slightly in front of your ears. Keep your arms parallel with palms facing inward, or press your palms together, whichever feels natural.
2. Exhale, bend your knees deeply so your thighs move toward parallel with the floor. Your knees will extend slightly past your toes, and your torso will lean forward over your thighs until your chest is roughly at a right angle with the tops of your legs.

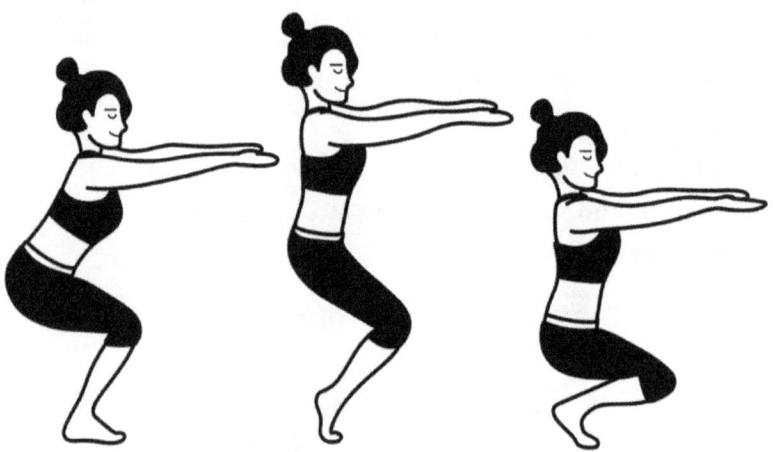

3. Keep your inner thighs parallel and press the tops of your thigh bones downward, anchoring toward your heels.
4. Firm your shoulder blades against your back. Lengthen your lower back by drawing your tailbone down and in toward your pubic bone.
5. To release, inhale and straighten your knees, lifting strongly through your arms. Exhale, lower your arms to your sides and return to Mountain Pose.

CHAIR POSE-TWISTED   Parivṛtta Utkaṭāsana

1. Begin in Mountain Pose, Tadasana, feet together, big toes touching. If you're newer to the practice, stand with feet hip-distance apart for more stability.
2. Inhale, raise your arms overhead, perpendicular to the floor. Exhale, bend your knees, and sink your hips, bringing your thighs as close to parallel with the floor as possible. Your knees may extend slightly beyond your toes; your torso will angle forward over your thighs. This is Chair Pose.
3. Lower your arms and bring your palms together at your chest. Exhale, twist your torso to the right, hooking your left elbow to the outside of your right thigh.
4. Shift your left hip back slightly, squaring off your hips once again. Bring your knees into alignment.

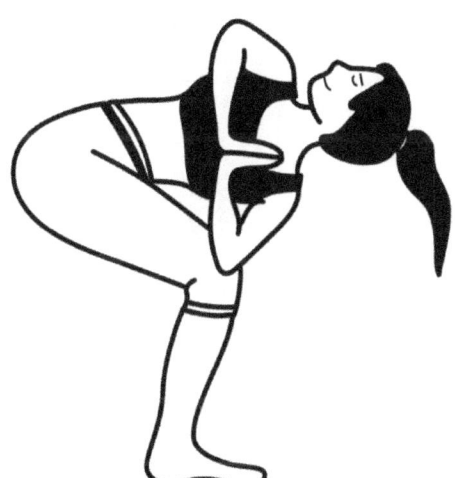

5. Press your upper left arm firmly into your thigh and draw your right shoulder blade into your back to rotate your chest to the right. To deepen the twist, extend both arms, right fingertips to the sky, left fingertips to the mat or block.

6. Turn your gaze upward. If your arms are extended, follow your top thumb with your eyes.
7. Drop your hips even lower. On each inhale, lengthen your spine. On each exhale, deepen your twist. Stack your shoulders and draw your thumbs toward your heart—then your heart toward your thumbs.
8. Keep your weight in your heels, pressing your feet firmly into the ground. Hold for up to one minute.
9. Inhale as you return to center, arms overhead in Chair Pose.
10. Exhale, straighten your legs and reach through your fingertips to return to Mountain Pose.
11. Repeat on the other side.

CHILD'S POSE — Balasana

1. Come onto your hands and knees. Spread your knees wide – about mat-width – while keeping the tops of your feet on the floor and your big toes touching.
2. Lower your belly between your thighs and bring your forehead to the floor. Let your shoulders, jaw, and eyes soften. If the floor doesn't feel comfortable, rest your forehead on a block or stack your hands into gentle fists.
3. Remain here for as long as you like. Soften your breath. Soften your body. Let the inhale and exhale become steady companions, bringing you home to yourself.

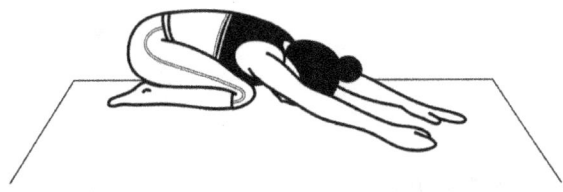

Note:

There's an energy point between the eyebrows that, when stimulated, helps activate the vagus nerve–supporting your "rest and digest" response. Finding a comfortable placement for your forehead can help access this calming effect.

Choose the arm position that best supports you:

Stretch your arms forward, palms down

Bring your arms back alongside your thighs, palms facing upward

Stretch arms forward with palms facing up for a shoulder release

Bend your elbows with palms together behind your neck and inch the elbows forward

Choose the variation that feels best for your body today. If your shoulders feel worked or fatigued, Option 2 offers welcome relief.

COBRA POSE — Bhujangasana

1. Begin on your belly, feet hip-distance apart, hands beside your ribs.
2. Extend your big toes straight back and press all 10 toenails into the mat to activate your quads.
3. Gently rotate your inner thighs toward the ceiling to broaden your lower back and create space across the sacrum.

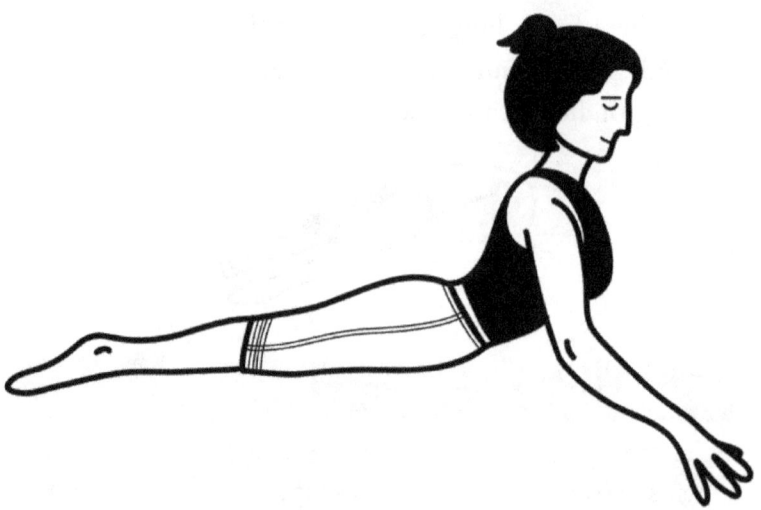

4. With light pressure through your palms, begin to lift your head and chest. Roll your shoulders back and down.
5. Keep the back of your neck long—lift through your sternum rather than straining the chin upward.
6. Begin to straighten your arms, keeping your elbows slightly bent and shoulders away from your ears. Let the lift originate from the heart, not from force.
7. To release, gently lower your chest back to the mat and rest.

The Yoga Postures

DOWNWARD FACING DOG
Adho Mukha Svanasana

1. Come to hands and knees positions. Align wrists under shoulders and knees under hips.
2. Curl your toes under. Press through your palms and lift your hips, straightening your legs into an inverted V shape.
3. Spread your fingers wide and root down through your fingertips and knuckles. Externally rotate the upper arms to broaden the collarbones.
4. Let your head hang heavy. Soften your neck. Glide your shoulder blades down your back, away from your ears.

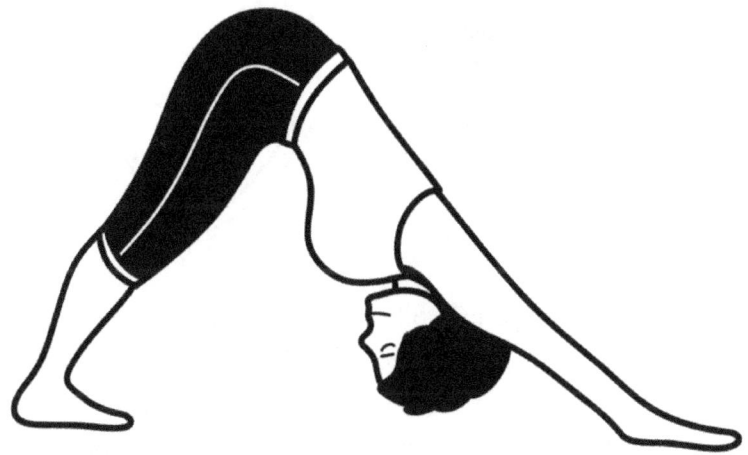

5. Engage your quadriceps to shift the workload from your arms. Let your thigh engagement support the lift.
6. Internally rotate your thighs, keep your tailbone high, and invite your heels toward the floor (no need to touch).
7. Check your form by moving forward into Plank Pose—your hand-to-foot distance should stay the same in both poses. Resist the urge to shorten the stance just to lower your heels.
8. To release, exhale and bend your knees, lowering gently back to hands and knees.

FETAL POSE — Pārśva Śavāsana

1. Sit on the floor with your knees bent and feet flat. Lean back onto your forearms.
2. Inhale, slowly extend your legs long on the mat, feet slightly apart, toes naturally turning outward.
3. Soften your lower back toward the floor. Lift your pelvis slightly, gently tuck your tailbone, and use your hand to guide your glutes away from the low back. Lower your pelvis. Rest briefly in Corpse Pose.

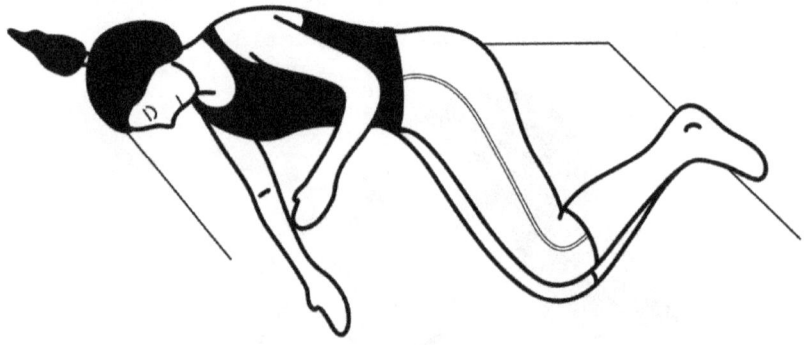

4. When ready, exhale and roll to one side. Extend your bottom arm and bend your knees. Rest your head on the extended arm.
5. Keep your eyes closed. Let your body soften. Let your breath guide you. Stay here for a few breaths—or as long as you need.

FOLDED BUTTERFLY POSE Baddha Koṇāsana

1. Begin in a seated position. Bring the soles of your feet together, letting your knees open out into a butterfly shape. Keep your feet a comfortable distance away from your pelvis.
2. Walk your hands forward as you hinge at the hips and fold. Allow your spine to round and release. Your hands may rest on your feet, reach forward, or land wherever feels natural.
3. Relax your spine and legs. Let gravity take over. Use props generously—a bolster, rolled blanket, or pillow under your hips or chest. If your neck feels strained, support your head by resting elbows on your thighs or a block.

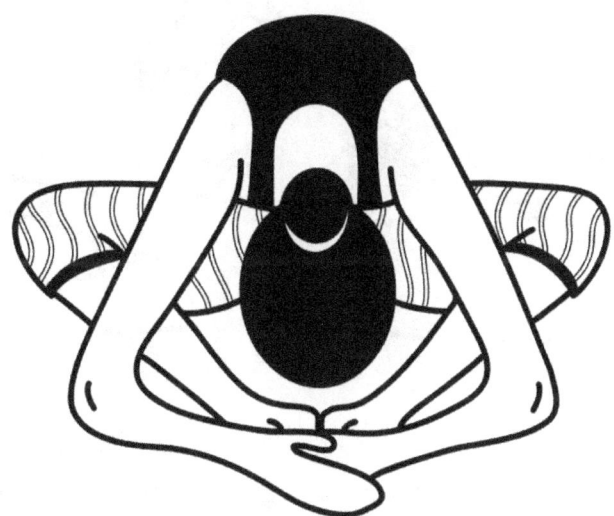

4. Stay here for 3-5 minutes. Soften into stillness. Let the breath rise and fall with ease.
5. To come out, press the floor away with your hands and slowly unroll your spine. Use your hands to gently bring your knees together. Lean back slightly, extend your legs forward, and rest with your arms behind you.

FORWARD BEND, SEATED Paschimottanasana

1. Sit with your legs extended straight in front of you. Gently press your sitting bones into the floor (or a folded blanket if needed). Draw your lower belly in and up. As you inhale, lengthen through your spine.
2. Exhale as you begin to fold forward, hinging from the hips. Only go as far as you can without rounding your back. Keep the movement long and lifted—not collapsed.

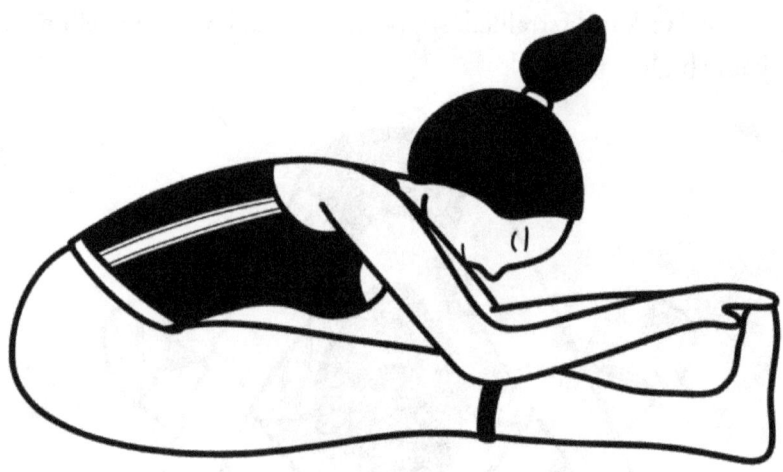

3. Lead with your belly and chest, not your forehead. Let the stretch ripple forward through your ribcage and chest. Use as many props as you need to stay supported. If you're folding deeper, allow your hands to glide along the floor or reach toward your feet. If accessible, wrap your peace fingers and thumbs around your big toes.
4. If you're using a strap, loop it around the soles of your feet and hold it with both hands. Keep your arms straight and elbows lifted away from the floor. Shoulders stay soft—don't let them climb toward your ears.

The Yoga Postures

5. With each inhale, gently lift your chest and lengthen your spine. With each exhale, fold forward a little more—hinging from the hips and staying connected to the breath. Walk your hands forward on the strap as your body invites you deeper into the stretch.
6. To come out, slowly walk your hands back toward your body. Let your hips glide back beneath you as the crown of your head reaches upward. Return to a tall spine, grounding through the sitting bones. Let each breath be an invitation—not a demand.
7. Send awareness into your hamstrings, your back, and the base of your spine. Soften. Settle. Stay with yourself.

FORWARD FOLD — Uttanasana

1. Begin in Mountain Pose (Tadasana) with your hands on your hips.
2. Exhale as you hinge at the hips, folding forward and lengthening through the front of your torso.
3. Bend your elbows and clasp opposite elbows with your hands. Let the crown of your head hang heavy. Root your heels into the floor as you lift your sit bones toward the ceiling. Gently rotate the tops of your thighs inward. Keep a soft bend in the knees—avoid locking them.
4. If your torso stays long and your knees remain comfortably straight, lower your hands to the mat beside your feet. Align your fingertips with your toes. If flexibility allows, bring your palms to the backs of your ankles.

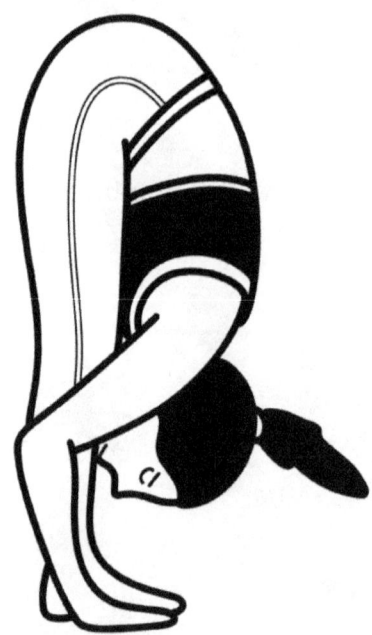

5. Engage your quads and draw them upward—this active engagement helps release the hamstrings.

6. Shift your weight slightly toward the balls of your feet while keeping your hips stacked over your ankles.
7. With every inhale, slightly lift and lengthen the torso. With every exhale, soften deeper into the fold. Let your neck relax and your head dangle freely.
8. Hold for up to one minute. To release, place your hands on your hips. Inhale, lengthen your spine, and rise with a flat back to return to Tadasana.

> **Note:**
>
> Let gravity be your guide. Let the breath be your release. Feel space open in the back of your legs—and let your thoughts pour out through the crown of your head.

FORWARD FOLD, WIDE-LEGGED
Prasarita Padottanasana

1. Begin in Mountain Pose facing the long edge of your mat. Step your feet wide—about 3 to 4 feet apart. Place your hands on your hips.
2. On an inhale, lift tall through your spine and chest. As you exhale, begin to fold forward from your hips, not your waist. Keep your spine long as you lower—pause if you feel your low back start to round.
3. Bring your hands to the floor, shoulder-width apart. If they don't reach, place them on blocks. Start to stretch your torso forward, then gradually deepen the fold—bringing your head closer to the mat.

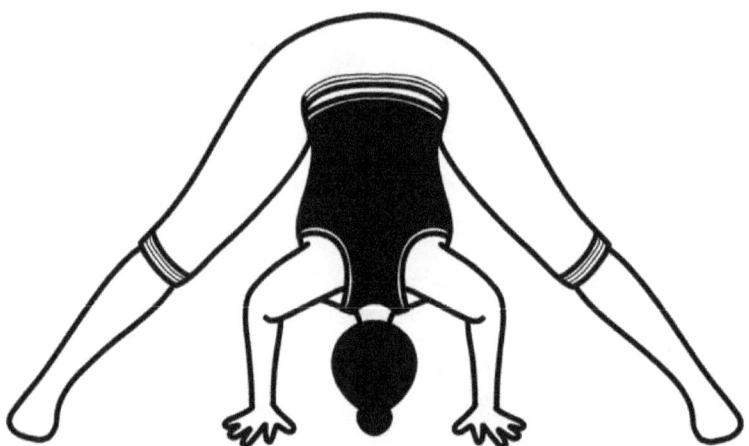

4. Ground through your feet and firm your thighs. Activate the inner legs. Let your sitting bones lift as you lengthen from your tailbone to the crown of your head.
5. Take several steady breaths here. With each inhale, lengthen your spine. With each exhale, soften deeper into the fold—without forcing.

The Yoga Postures

6. When you're ready to come out, ground into your feet, straighten your arms, and slowly rise on an inhale. Step your feet back together and return to Mountain Pose. Pause and feel the shift.

> **Note:**
>
> The wider your stance, the more space you'll have to fold—but not too wide. If you feel unstable, shorten your stance slightly.
>
> If there's tightness in your back or legs, bend your knees as much as needed to stay safe and grounded.
>
> Send your breath to the hamstrings and inner thighs. Let the exhale create ease in your spine.

GARLAND POSE — Malasana

1. Stand with your feet about mat's width apart. Bend your knees and begin to lower your hips toward the floor into a squat. Let your toes naturally turn out slightly—but avoid overdoing it. Eventually, you're working toward keeping the feet closer to parallel.
2. Bring your upper arms inside your knees and bend your elbows, pressing your palms together at your heart center. Let your thumbs gently touch your sternum to help keep the chest lifted.
3. Engage by pressing your arms into your thighs—and your thighs right back into your arms. This counter-pressure helps you stay lifted and strong.
4. Keep your spine long, your tailbone reaching toward the floor, and your shoulders relaxed away from your ears. Let your breath flow freely. Close your eyes if it helps you tune in.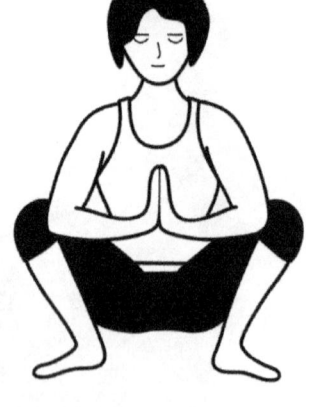
5. Stay here for five slow breaths. Let each exhale soften your hips toward the earth. When you're ready to release, straighten your legs and return to standing—or flow directly into a forward fold if that feels good.
6. Repeat the sequence three times to build warmth and deepen your squat. Inhale to prepare. Exhale to squat. Let this become a rhythm your body remembers.

Note:

If your heels lift off the ground, try placing a rolled blanket or folded mat underneath them for support. Over time, your flexibility will increase, but don't force it. Ease opens more than effort does.

GODDESS POSE — Utkata Konasana

1. Stand with your feet wider than shoulder-width apart—a strong, grounded stance. You'll want enough distance to bend your knees easily, but not so much that you lose stability.
2. Turn your toes outward, pointing toward the corners of your mat. Begin to bend your knees and lower into a squat.
3. Tuck your tailbone, draw your belly button up and in, and externally rotate your thighs. Keep your spine long and shoulders relaxed as you settle deeper.

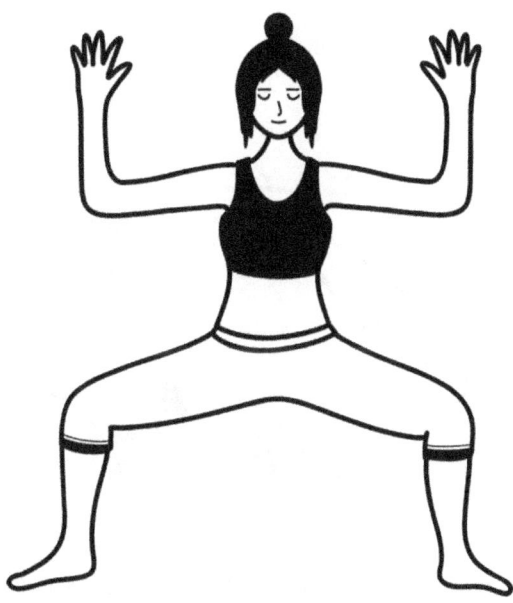

4. Make sure your knees stay stacked over your ankles. If your body allows, aim to bring your thighs parallel to the floor.
5. Place your arms wherever they feel strong and natural. Traditionally, bend your elbows to form a goalpost shape, fingers spread wide like you're claiming your space.
6. Breathe here for 4–8 deep breaths. Sink low. Stay tall. Stand in your power. Be the Goddess.

HALF BOW POSE — Ardha Dhanurasana

1. Lie flat on your belly. Keep your chin on the mat and arms resting at your sides, palms facing up.
2. Exhale as you bend your right knee, drawing your heel as close to your glutes as you can.
3. Reach your right hand back and take hold of your right ankle—not the top of your foot. Wrap your fingers around the ankle; your thumb stays off. Keep your toes pointed.
4. As you inhale, lift your heel away from your glutes, creating resistance in your arm. At the same time, lift your head, chest, and thigh off the mat. Anchor your opposite arm and leg firmly into the floor.

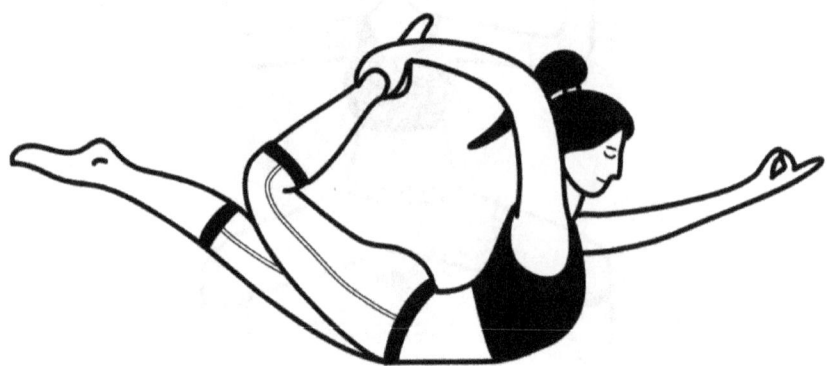

5. Let your shoulders rotate open naturally and draw your tailbone down to stabilize and deepen the stretch.
6. Feel your chest expand and the front of your body energize as you open into the pose. Breathe into the space you're creating.
7. Exhale to release. Lower your thigh, chest, and head back to the mat. Gently let go of your ankle and return your hand to your side.
8. Pause. Breathe. Then switch to the other side.

HALF CAMEL POSE — Ardha Ustrasana

1. From Child's Pose or Hero Pose, rise up onto both knees, placing them hip-width apart. Rest your palms on your sacrum, fingers pointing down.
2. Inhale and press your knees into the mat as you lift through the crown of your head, lengthening your spine.
3. Exhale and press your hips forward. Squeeze your glutes and inner thighs for support as you begin to arch back, using your hands for stability.
4. Gently reach your right hand toward your right heel. If your hand doesn't reach, no worries—keep it on your sacrum for now.
5. Inhale and extend your left arm up and back behind you. If it feels safe for your neck, let your head drop back completely. Hold for 3–6 deep breaths.
6. To come out of the pose, bring both hands to your sacrum. Inhale slowly as you lift your torso upright—let your head and neck be the last to rise. Pause here. Breathe. Reset.
7. Repeat on the other side.

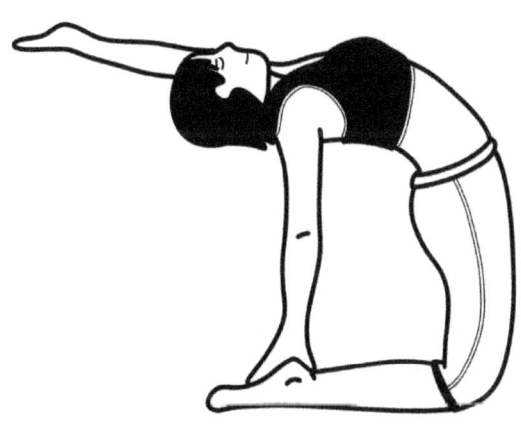

Note:

Every movement in this pose should be slow, steady, and deliberate. Rushing may lead to lightheadedness. Let intention guide the way.

HALF FROG POSE — Ardha Bhekasana

1. Lie on your belly with your forearms resting on the mat, parallel to each other. Find length in your spine and gently draw your shoulders away from your ears.
2. Exhale, bend your right knee, and bring your foot toward your bottom. Reach back with your right hand and grasp the top of your foot. Let your fingers point forward and your elbow reach toward the sky.
3. To deepen the pose, extend your left arm forward on the mat. Keep your breath steady and calm. With each inhale, soften your belly to the floor; with each exhale, release tension where you feel it most.
4. After a few full breaths, gently release your foot and return your leg to the mat. Take a grounding inhale and prepare for the other side.

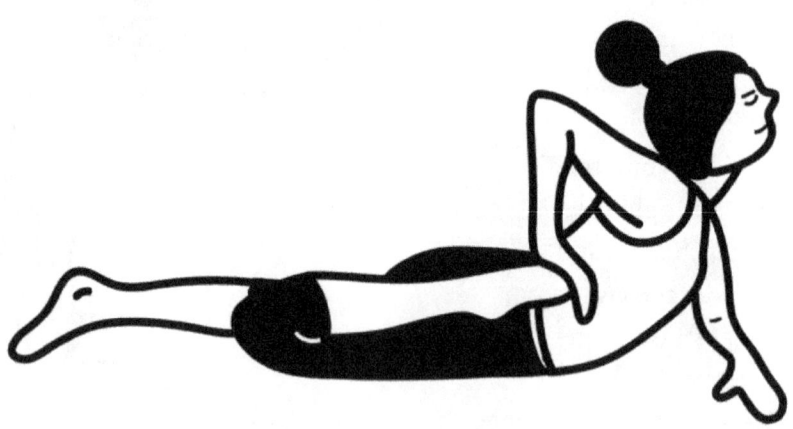

5. Exhale, bend your left knee and reach your left hand back to hold your foot—again, fingers pointing forward, elbow reaching upward.

6. Straighten your right arm along the floor to balance the stretch. Breathe into the front of your thigh and the openness across your chest.
7. When you're ready, gently let go of your foot and return to lying flat on your mat. Pause here and notice the sensation shift in your body.

> **Note:**
> This pose is powerful for opening the quads, hips, and chest—areas that often hold tension and restrict circulation. Let your breath guide your body's ability to release.

HALF LORD OF THE FISHES
Ardha Matsyendrasan

1. Begin seated in Easy Pose (Sukhasana). Cross your right knee over your left, bringing your feet alongside your hips. Lift your right knee and place the sole of your right foot on the floor outside your left knee.
2. Place your right hand on the floor just behind your right hip for support. Sit evenly on both sitting bones.
3. Inhale and reach your left arm toward the ceiling, lengthening through the spine.
4. Exhale, bring your left elbow to the outside of your right knee. Press your elbow and knee together to create gentle resistance.
5. Turn your head to the right, gazing softly past your shoulder. Keep your neck easy and relaxed—no strain.
6. Stay here for several breaths. Inhale to lift and lengthen the spine. Exhale to gently deepen the twist. Let your breath guide the rotation without forcing it.
7. To come out, inhale to unwind, lifting your right arm. Exhale, return to center with awareness.

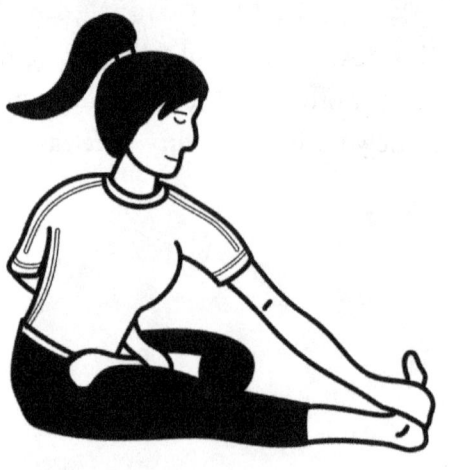

Note:

This spinal twist stimulates digestion, restores spinal mobility, and supports emotional release. With each exhale, send your breath into the base of your spine and invite in spaciousness.

HALF PIGEON POSE
Eka Pada Rajakapotasana

1. From Downward Facing Dog, lift your right leg into the air for a gentle Down Dog Split. Pause to stretch and lengthen your leg fully.
2. Bend your right knee and bring the leg forward, as if stepping into a lunge. Instead of placing your foot between your hands, guide your right knee to the floor, just outside your right wrist. Your right shin may angle back toward your left hip or be more parallel to the front of the mat—let your body decide.
3. Lower your left knee to the mat. Extend your left leg straight behind you, with your toes pointing back. Take a quick glance behind to make sure the left foot is aligned and your leg is straight.
4. Square your hips toward the front of the mat. Use props—a folded blanket or block under your right hip—to bring balance and stability.

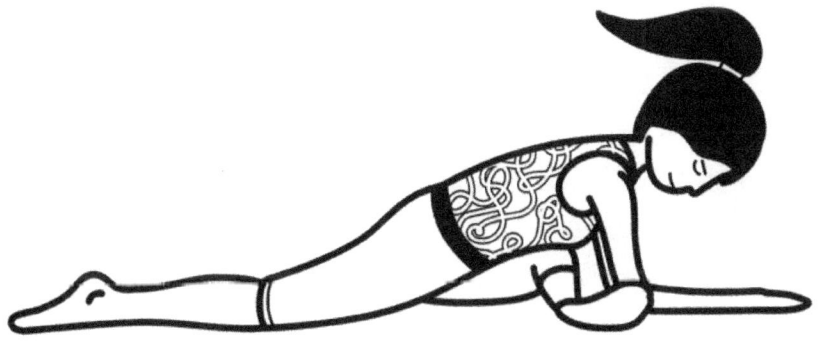

5. If you feel grounded and steady, begin to fold forward, bringing your forearms or forehead to the mat, reaching toward the earth.
6. Let your hips stay square, allowing gravity to do the work. If the stretch feels too intense, support yourself with additional props.

7. Stay for several breaths, inhaling to create space in the hips, and exhaling to soften into the posture. Notice where tension lingers and send your breath there.
8. To release, place your hands under your shoulders, curl your left toes, and step back into Downward Facing Dog.

This is a pose of surrender. Stay with it. Breathe into the edges of resistance, and trust your body to meet you where you are.

HALFWAY LIFT — Ardha Uttanasana

1. Begin in Standing Forward Fold (Uttanasana), with your hands or fingertips on the floor beside your feet. If the floor feels far away, place your hands on your shins or use yoga blocks beneath your palms.
2. Inhale as you lift your torso halfway up, straightening your elbows and lengthening your spine.
3. Lift your collarbones and sternum away from the floor. Reach the crown of your head forward and your tailbone back, creating space from end to end.
4. Press your fingertips or palms into the floor (or blocks) to support your lift. If your back rounds, bend your knees or adjust your hand placement until your spine is flat.
5. Engage your quadriceps by lifting them toward the ceiling. Keep a slight bend in the knees and root your weight into the balls of your feet, aligning your hips over your ankles.
6. With each inhale, lengthen your spine. With each exhale, soften your jaw and shoulders.
7. Hold the pose for up to one minute. To release, exhale as you fold forward into Uttanasana.

Note:

Think of this pose as a pause. A reset. A moment of length and strength before you return to the flow.

HAPPY BABY POSE — Ananda Balasana

1. Lie flat on your back. As you exhale, bend your knees into your belly.
2. Inhale, reach your hands up and grab the outsides of your feet. If that's not accessible, loop a strap or belt over each foot instead.
3. Open your knees wider than your torso, then draw them up toward your armpits. Exhale and soften.

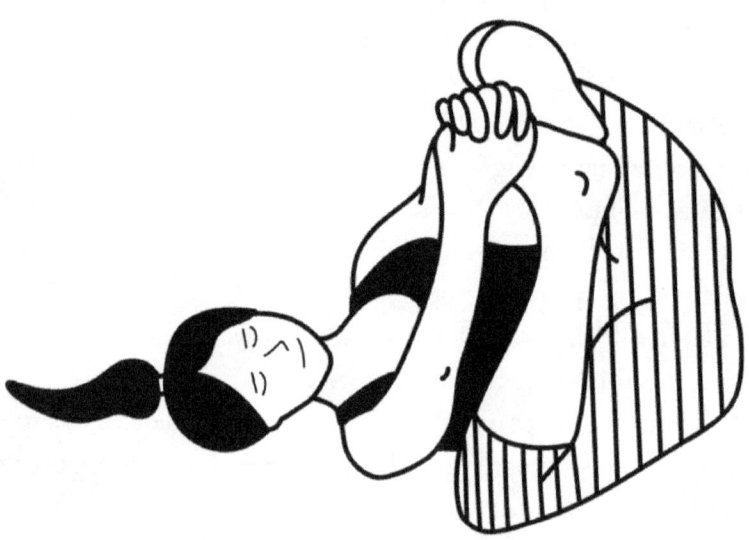

4. Stack each ankle directly over the knee so your shins are vertical—flex your feet like you mean it.
5. Gently press your feet into your hands (or straps) as you pull down—creating just the right amount of resistance.
6. Rock, sway, stillness—find the movement that feels right for your body.

HERO POSE — Virasana

1. Begin in Tabletop Pose on your hands and knees. Slowly lift your torso upright so that your weight shifts fully onto your shins and knees.
2. Bring your knees closer together, then separate your feet slightly wider than hip-distance apart. Keep the tops of your feet pressing down into the mat.
3. Lower your hips back between your heels. Sit directly on the mat—or on a block, bolster, or rolled blanket for support. Take your time. There's no rush.

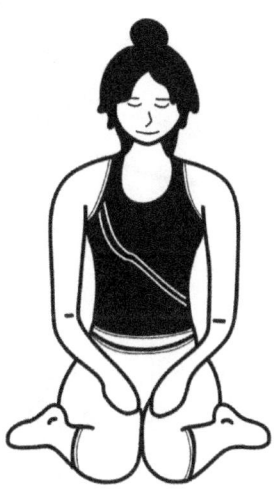

4. Use your hands to gently roll the flesh of your calves outward to make space. Draw your navel in and up, ground through your sitting bones, and lengthen through the crown of your head.
5. Close your eyes or soften your gaze. Breathe here for 5 to 10 breaths. Let your spine lift and your hips settle.
6. To come out, place your hands on the mat in front of you, lift your hips, and return to Tabletop Pose.
7. Sway your hips side to side or take any gentle movement your body asks for to release the knees and ankles.

HIGH PLANK — Kumbhakasana

1. From Downward-Facing Dog, shift your torso forward until it's parallel with the ground. Stack your shoulders directly over your wrists, arms strong and vertical.
2. Spread your fingers wide and root down firmly through the bases of your index fingers and thumbs. Draw your outer arms inward as you broaden across your shoulder blades.

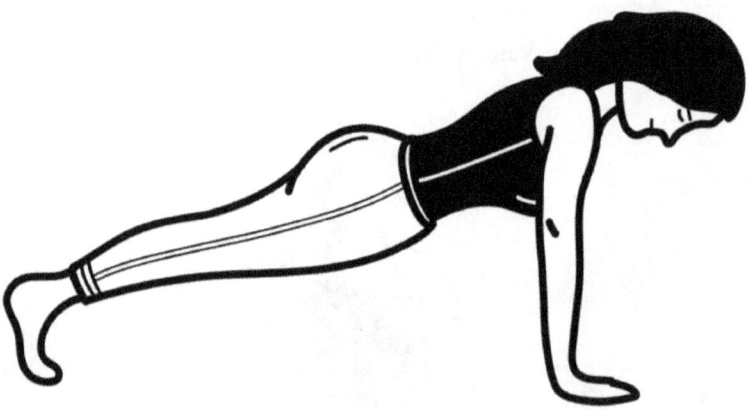

3. Press your chest forward while reaching your heels back. Engage your legs and core, supporting your pelvis so that it stays lifted—not sagging or arching.
4. Keep your gaze straight down, lengthening through the back of your neck. Your body should feel like one strong, connected line from head to heel.
5. Hold the pose with steady breath—long and even. Start with what feels manageable, and gradually work your way up to a 60-second hold over time.

HORIZON'S LUNGE
Parivrtta Anjaneyasan Variation

1. Begin in a low runner's lunge, with your front knee bent and stacked over the ankle. Extend the arm on the same side as your front leg forward—fingers spread wide, palm facing inward. Your other hand is rooted to the mat inside your front thigh for support. Gaze forward.
2. From here, lift your extended arm toward the sky, still on the same side as your front leg. Keep your supporting palm grounded—either inside or outside the front thigh, depending on what feels best in your body. Gaze upward, or down to the earth if your neck is sensitive.
3. Reach your top arm even higher, then begin to sweep it back, rotating from the shoulder. As you do, roll onto the pinky-edge sides of both feet, flexing them to protect your joints.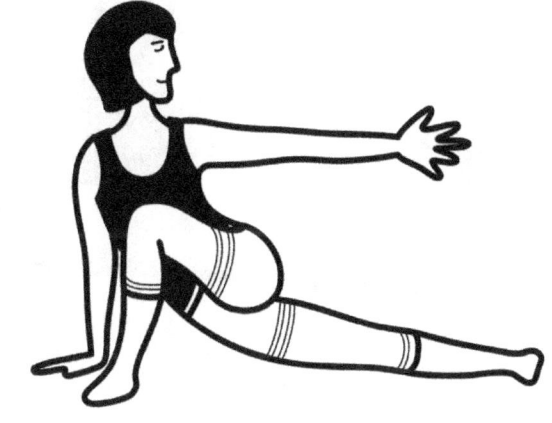
4. Firm your extended leg, and sink your hips low—rooting down into the earth. Your top arm extends parallel to the floor, palm facing behind you. Send your breath into your side body and lengthen through your fingertips.
5. Gently bring your top hand back to the mat, close your hips, and return to tabletop position.
6. Take a breath. Repeat on the opposite side.

KNEES TO CHEST — Apanasana

1. Begin by lying on your back with your arms and legs extended, palms facing up.
2. As you exhale, draw both knees in toward your chest. Wrap your arms around your shins. If it's available to you, cross your forearms and clasp opposite elbows.
3. Keep your entire back connected to the mat. Soften your shoulders and let your shoulder blades melt down toward your waist. Broaden gently across your collarbones.

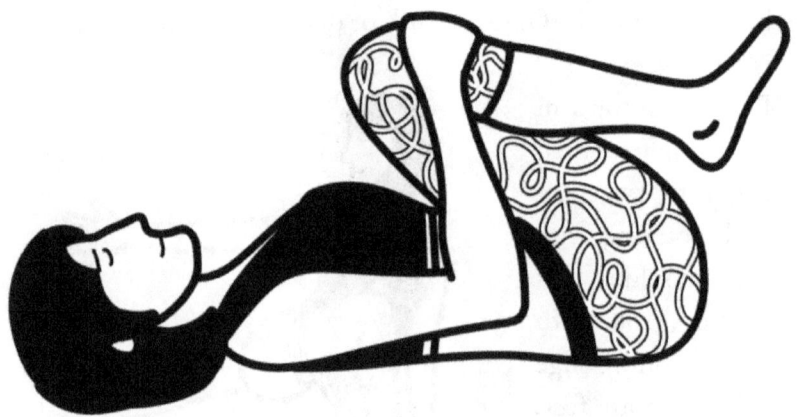

4. Lengthen your spine by drawing your tailbone and sacrum down toward the mat. Feel your lower back settle. If it feels good, begin to rock slowly side to side or front to back, allowing a gentle massage of the spine.
5. Tuck your chin slightly and let your gaze follow the midline of your body. Stay soft in the jaw and forehead.
6. Hold here for up to one minute, breathing smoothly and evenly. When you're ready, exhale to release your arms and extend your legs along the mat into rest.

LEGS UP THE WALL POSE — Viparita Karani

1. Sit on the floor with one hip close to a wall. Gently lower your shoulders and head to the ground, lying on your side.
2. As you roll onto your back, sweep your legs up the wall. Your feet can be hip-distance apart or positioned however feels most natural for your body.
3. Adjust by scooting your hips closer to the wall, but don't worry if your tailbone doesn't touch it. Let comfort—not perfection—guide your position.

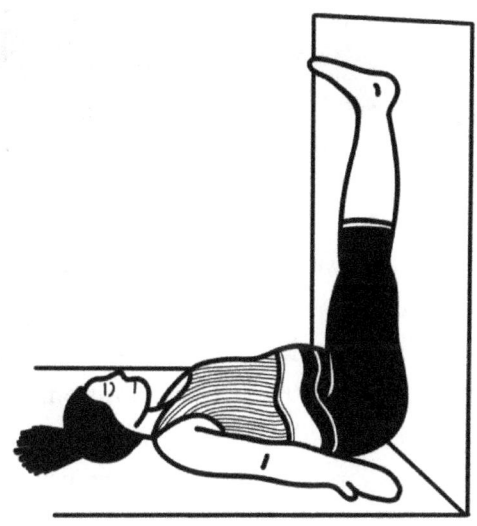

4. Rest your arms by your sides, palms turned up. Allow your shoulders to melt into the mat.
5. Relax fully. Let the weight of your legs rest against the wall, and feel your thigh bones gently release into your hip sockets. Notice your spine lengthening. Let gravity do the work.
6. Stay here for several minutes, breathing slowly and softly. When you're ready to come out, bend your knees and roll to one side. Pause here for a few breaths, then press up gently with your hands to return to a seated position.

LIZARD POSE — Utthan Pristhasana

1. Begin in Downward Facing Dog. Take a deep inhale.
2. As you exhale, step your right foot to the outside of your right hand. Bring the foot all the way forward so that your toes line up with your fingertips. Your knee should be bent at about 90 degrees and stacked directly over your ankle. Let your toes angle out slightly, around 45 degrees.

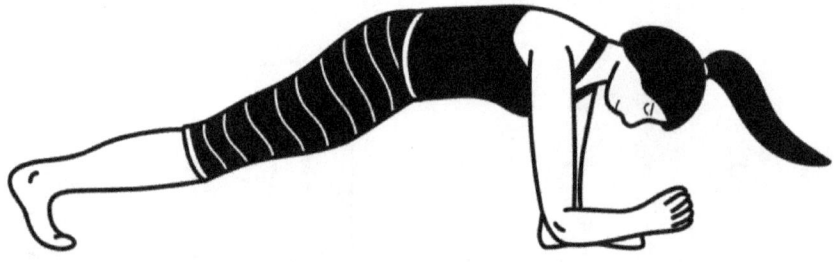

3. Inhale and begin to lower your elbows toward the floor, bringing your forearms parallel and flat on the mat. If your body needs support, place a block under your forearms.
4. Keep your head in a neutral, relaxed position. Exhale and press firmly through your back heel—this will activate your left leg and help keep your hips supported and lifted. Stay here for 5 full, deep breaths.
5. To come out of the pose, exhale and gently straighten your arms, placing your palms under your shoulders. Inhale as you step back to Downward Facing Dog. Pause here and take a few slow, reset breaths.
6. When you're ready, repeat on the left side.

LOCUST POSE — Salabhasana

1. Begin on your belly with your feet together and arms extended back behind you, palms facing down. Rest your forehead or chin on the mat. As you exhale, gently press your pubic bone into the floor to lengthen your lower back and draw your belly button in toward your spine.
2. Activate your legs—especially your quads, the muscles on the front of your thighs. Inhale and lift your head, chest, arms, and legs off the mat.

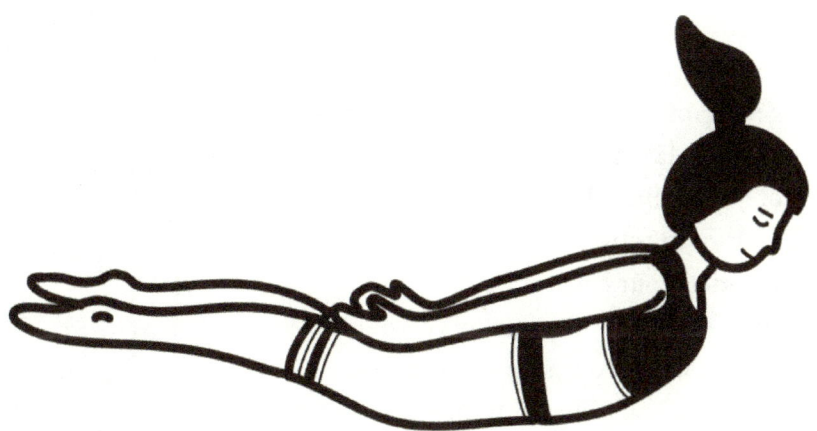

3. Draw your shoulder blades together as you lift, rolling your shoulders up and back. Imagine someone gently pulling your hands behind you to help you rise a little higher.
4. Your feet can be together or hip-width apart—whatever feels best in your body. Draw them toward the midline without straining. Hold the pose for 5 deep, steady breaths.
5. When you're ready to come out, exhale as you slowly lower back down with control. Rest briefly, then repeat the pose two more times if it feels good for your body.

MOUNTAIN POSE — Tadasana

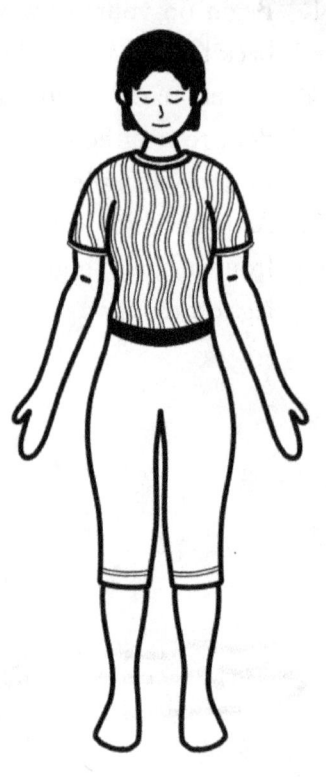

1. Stand tall with your big toes touching. Lift all ten toes, fan them out wide, then set them back down to create a stable, grounded base. If your ankles knock together uncomfortably, separate your heels slightly. Let your feet and calves root firmly into the earth.
2. Engage your quads—the muscles on the front of your thighs—and lift your kneecaps. Rotate your thighs gently inward to widen your sitting bones. Maintain the natural curves of your spine. Draw your belly in slightly to activate your core.
3. Broaden your collarbones and stack your shoulders directly over your pelvis. Shrug your shoulders upward your ears, then roll them back and down so your shoulder blades glide along your spine. Let your arms hang softly with a gentle bend at the elbows and your palms facing forward.
4. Keep your neck long. Your chin should be neutral—not tucked or lifted. Imagine the crown of your head reaching up toward the sky.
5. Once you're aligned, breathe. Hold the pose for 5 to 10 breaths, feeling strength and steadiness through your entire body.

PUPPY POSE — Uttana Shishosana

1. Begin in tabletop pose, with your shoulders stacked above your wrists and your hips aligned above your knees. Tuck your toes under rather than pointing them.
2. Keeping your hips over your knees, begin to slowly walk your hands forward, extending your arms long in front of you.

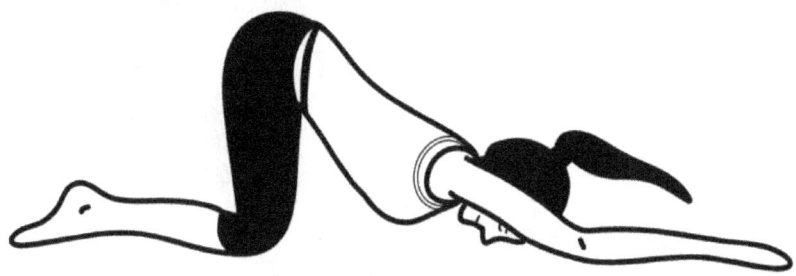

3. Depending on your comfort and neck mobility, rest your forehead on the mat, on a block, or bring your gaze forward to allow your chin to rest gently on the floor.
4. To deepen the stretch through your spine, chest, and shoulders, press your palms into the mat and isometrically draw your hips back. Feel the lengthening from your fingertips to your tailbone.
5. Hold the pose for up to one minute. When you're ready to release, gently shift your hips back into Child's Pose and reconnect with your breath.

RABBIT POSE — Sasangasana

1. From a kneeling position, reach your hands back and firmly grasp your heels. Begin to draw your forehead in toward your knees as much as possible, creating a deep forward curl.

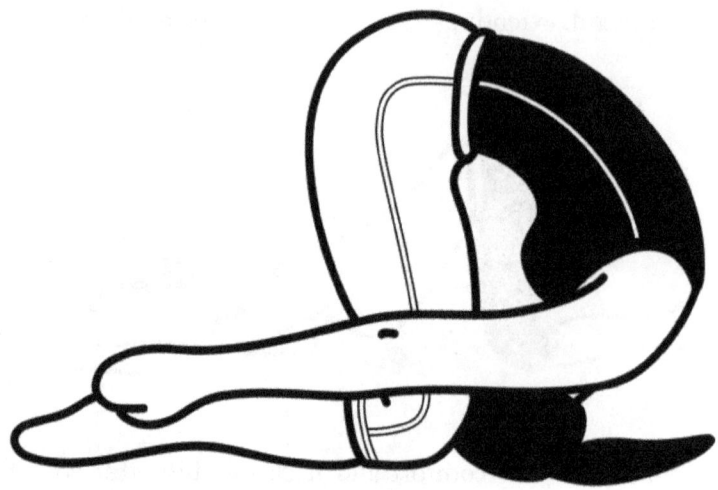

2. Inhale as you gently lift your hips off your heels, slowly rolling onto the crown of your head. Keep your grip strong and steady. Stretch your arms back along your heels as you lift, creating length in the spine. Breathe deeply, feeling the stretch through your back and the gentle traction in your neck—without straining.
3. Hold the pose for 30 to 60 seconds, breathing steadily.
4. Exhale to lower your hips back to your heels and gently release your hands. Extend your arms forward and rest in Child's Pose to soften and reset.

RECLINED BOUND ANGLE
Supta Baddha Koṇāsana

1. Lie down comfortably on your back with your legs extended and arms at your sides, palms facing up. Support your back with a blanket, bolster, or block—whatever feels best for your body today.
2. Bend your knees and bring the soles of your feet together, letting the outer edges of your feet rest on the mat. Allow your knees to fall open, supported by gravity. Use a rolled blanket or block under each knee for extra support—there should be no tension or effort in keeping the legs in position.

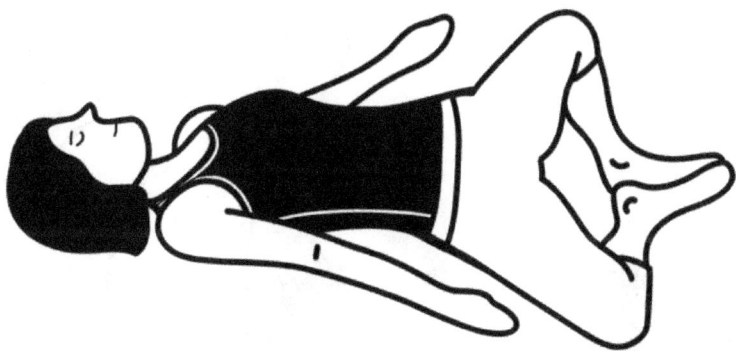

3. Tune in to your body. If your hips or groin feel tight, slide your feet further away from your pelvis. If you're feeling more open, draw your feet closer in to deepen the stretch.
4. Relax your shoulders down and away from your ears. Let your back body soften and melt into the mat or prop beneath you. Stay here for 1–5 minutes, depending on what feels good.
5. To come out of the pose, place your palms on your outer thighs and gently draw your legs together. Bring the soles of your feet flat to the mat, then hug your knees to your chest and rock side to side to release the low back.

RECLINED FIGURE 4 POSE
Supta Kapotāsana

1. Begin lying on your back with knees bent and feet flat on the floor, close to your hips. Settle your spine into the mat.
2. Lift your right leg and bring the knee toward your chest. Then cross your right ankle over your left thigh, just above the knee. Flex your right foot to protect your knee joint.
3. If you feel a strong enough stretch here—stay. Otherwise, thread your right hand between your legs and clasp your hands behind your left thigh, drawing it gently toward your chest.

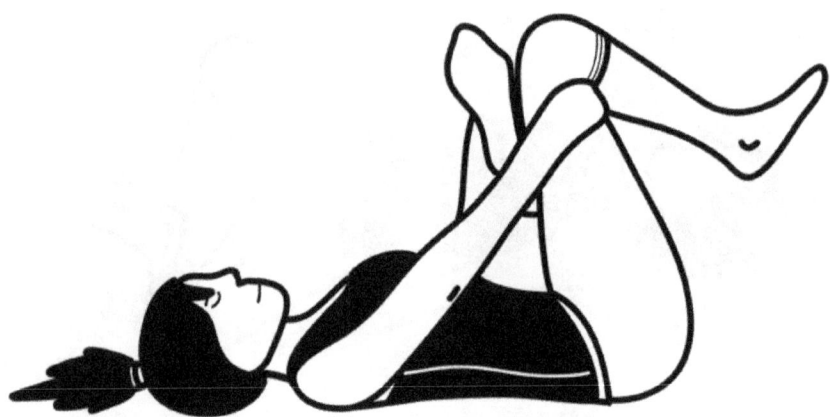

4. Keep your shoulders grounded, jaw soft, and gaze upward. Avoid straining—this is about ease and awareness. Let your breath guide the release. Breathe deeply, encouraging the hips to soften on every exhale.
5. Stay here for a few rounds of breath. When ready, uncross your legs and return both feet to the floor.
6. Repeat on the other side, moving with the same intention and presence.

RECLINING EAGLE TWIST
Supta Parivṛtta Garuḍāsana

1. Lie down on your back and hug your knees in toward your chest. Cross your right leg over your left. If it feels good in your body, hook your right foot behind your left calf—but only if it's accessible without strain.
2. Let your knees drop to the left, allowing gravity to guide them down. Don't force them—this is about release, not resistance.
3. Open your arms out wide into a goal post shape. Soften your shoulders toward the mat and let your heart feel supported.

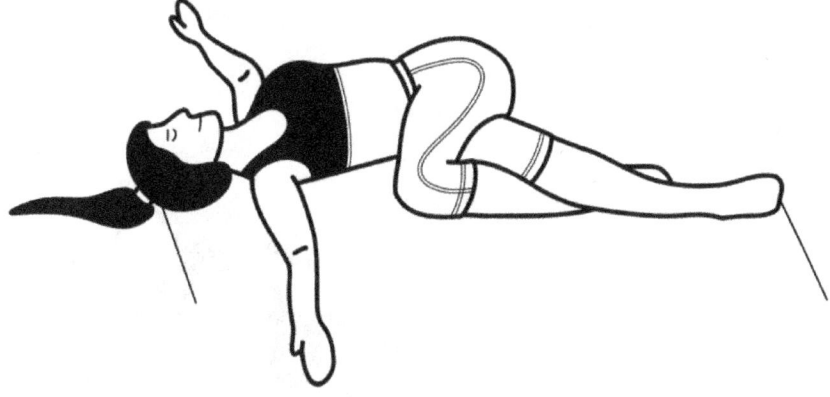

4. Gently turn your head to the right, gazing over your shoulder—only if your neck feels comfortable.
5. Stay for 5 deep breaths, allowing your breath to travel down your spine and into the twist. Let your exhales help you melt more deeply into the pose.
6. To come out, return to center, uncross your legs, and switch sides when you're ready.

RUNNER'S LUNGE
Utthita Ashwa Sanchalanasana

1. From tabletop position, step your right foot forward between your hands. Stack your knee over your ankle. Tuck your back toes under and begin to straighten your back leg.
2. Press your palms, fingertips, or fists into the ground to lift your chest and the crown of your head upward. Roll your shoulders back and shine your chest forward. Gaze straight ahead, keeping your chin parallel to the floor.
3. Extend your back leg by pressing the heel toward the floor and reaching the back of your knee toward the ceiling. Let your hips sink gently downward. Breathe deeply and hold the pose for 2–6 breaths.

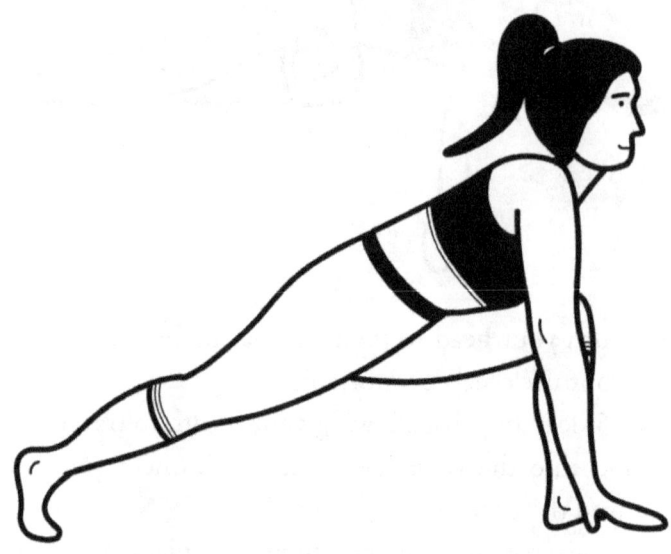

4. When you're ready to release, lower your back knee and either slide the front leg back into tabletop or step back into downward-facing dog.

5. Repeat on the other side, giving equal attention and breath to both legs.

> **Note:**
>
> In Low Runner's Lunge, your hands remain grounded with fingertips tented or palms pressing.
>
> In High Runner's Lunge, your arms extend overhead, palms facing one another, reaching tall.

SEATED STAFF POSE — Dandasana

1. Sit tall with your legs extended straight in front of you, feet together. Place your hands beside your hips, fingertips pressing into the floor.
2. Flex your feet, pressing out through your heels. Engage your thighs and actively root your sitting bones down into the earth. Draw your lower belly in and up to support your spine.

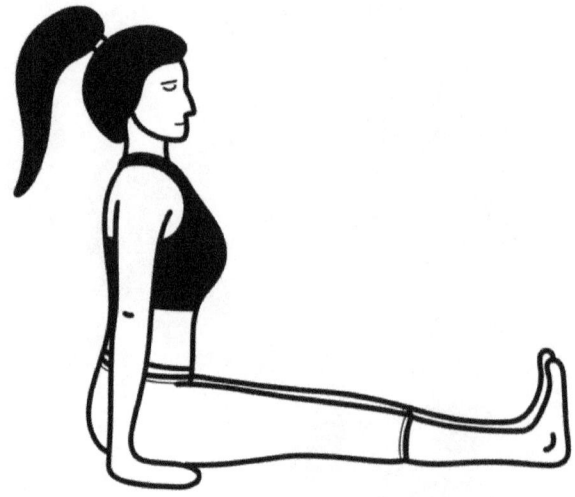

3. Slide your shoulder blades up, then back and down along your spine. Let the bottom tips of your shoulder blades hug toward each other. Keep your collarbones broad, your chin slightly tucked, and your neck soft and long.
4. Stay here for 5 to 15 breaths, keeping your core engaged and your posture active.

Note:

This pose may look simple—but it asks you to sit with strength, awareness, and grace.

SEATED SUN SALUTATIONS
Upavistha Surya Namaskar

1. Sit cross-legged in the center of your mat—or choose hero pose if that feels better in your body. Make sure you're sitting tall with a lifted spine and freedom to move your arms.
2. Bring your hands together in front of your heart, thumb knuckles lightly pressing against your sternum. Let that gentle pressure lift your heart forward.

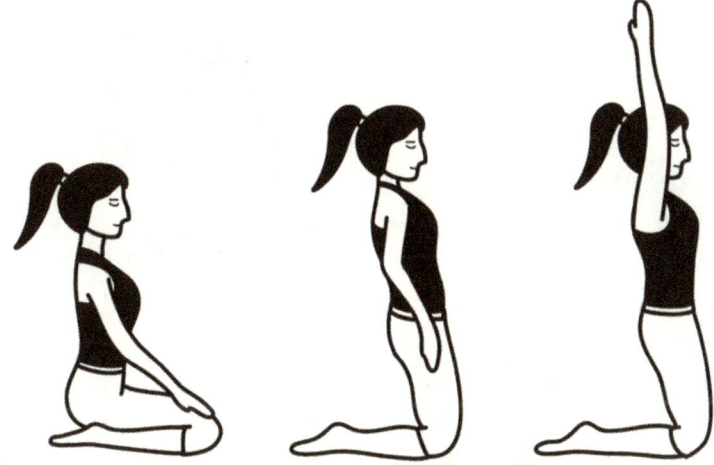

3. Draw your chin away from your chest. Inhale deeply as you sweep your arms up to the sky, gaze lifting toward your fingertips. Open your arms wide as you reach—lift from the shoulders, elongate the spine, and breathe into the stretch.
4. Exhale slowly as you bring your palms back together and lower them to your heart, drawing the energy back in. Drop your chin slightly as you return to a neutral, grounded gaze.
5. Inhale, rise again. Reach wide and tall.
6. Exhale, come back down.
7. Repeat this flowing motion for several cycles, matching breath to movement.

SEATED TORSO CIRCLES — Sufi Grinds

1. Sit cross-legged with your spine tall and upright. Gently close your eyes. Place your hands on your knees and begin to move your spine in large, slow circles around your pelvis.
2. Inhale as you rotate forward, expanding through the chest. Exhale as you round back, drawing your navel toward your spine. Let your breath guide your movement.

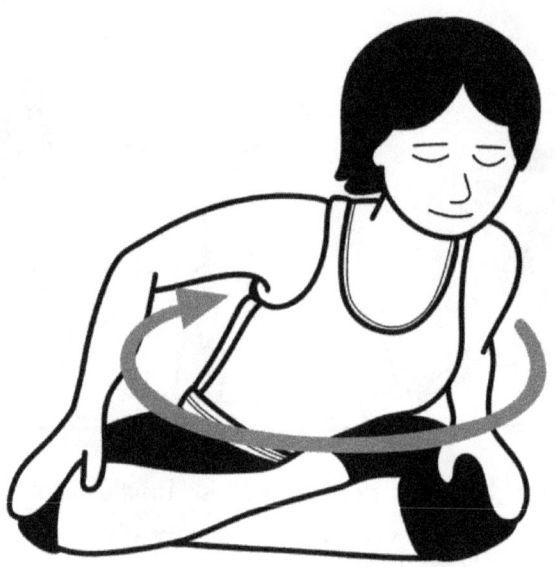

3. Make the circles as big and expressive or as small and subtle as you'd like. There's no right or wrong—this is your time to explore and feel into your body.
4. Continue in one direction for about a minute, then reverse and circle the other way for another minute. Let the motion loosen the spine, hips, and waist.

SEATED TWIST — Parivrtta Sukhasana

1. Begin seated with your legs extended in front of you. Cross your legs at the shins, bringing each foot beneath the opposite knee. This is Easy Pose (Sukhasana). If your hips are tight, sit on a bolster or block for support.
2. Ground evenly through your sitting bones. Sit tall with a long spine and relaxed shoulders. Let your neck soften and your legs settle naturally.
3. Place your right hand behind you for support. On an exhale, bring your left hand to the outside of your right knee and gently begin to twist to the right.
4. Inhale to lengthen your spine; exhale to deepen the twist. Let your gaze follow, turning gently over your right shoulder.

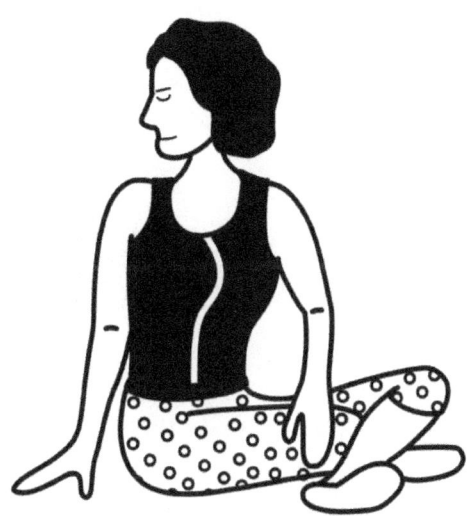

5. Avoid pushing or forcing. Keep your collarbones broad and your shoulders relaxed. Stay upright and centered—don't lean forward to chase the twist.
6. Hold here for up to 10 breaths, using each inhale to create space and each exhale to gently settle deeper.
7. Exhale as you unwind back to center. Switch the cross of your legs, and repeat the twist on the other side.

SPHINX POSE — Salamba Bhujangasana

1. Begin lying on your belly, legs extended long behind you, feet together. Rest your forearms flat on the floor, elbows directly under your shoulders, and your chin touching the mat.
2. As you inhale, press firmly through your forearms and begin to lift your head and chest. Keep your neck long, aligned with your spine.
3. Engage your quads and glutes, drawing the kneecaps up and pressing the pubic bone into the mat to ground and stabilize your lower body.

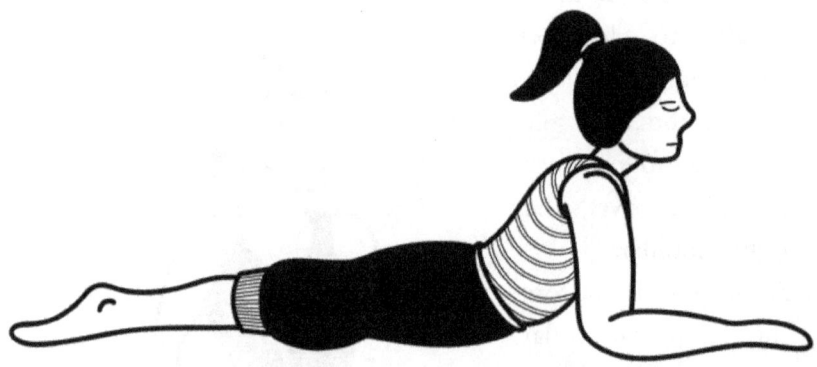

4. Keep your elbows hugging in toward your sides. Use your arms to gently lift your heart higher while keeping the shoulders soft and rolled back. Press your chest forward and draw your chin inward slightly, lengthening the back of your neck.
5. If it feels safe, lift your gaze slightly or direct it toward the space between your eyebrows—the third eye point.
6. Hold for 2–6 breaths, breathing deeply into the front body and noticing any sensations rising in the spine or pelvis.
7. To come out, exhale slowly, lowering your chest and head back to the mat. Turn your head to one side, bring your arms alongside your body, and allow yourself to fully rest.

STAR POSE — Utthita Tadasana

1. Begin in Mountain Pose (Tadasana) at the top of your mat. Stand tall with your feet about hip-width apart and your spine elongated. Place your hands on your hips.
2. Step your feet out wide—as wide as feels comfortable—and let your toes angle out slightly toward the corners of your mat.
3. Extend both arms out to the sides at shoulder height, forming a star shape. Your feet and wrists should align roughly with each other, creating a sense of spaciousness.

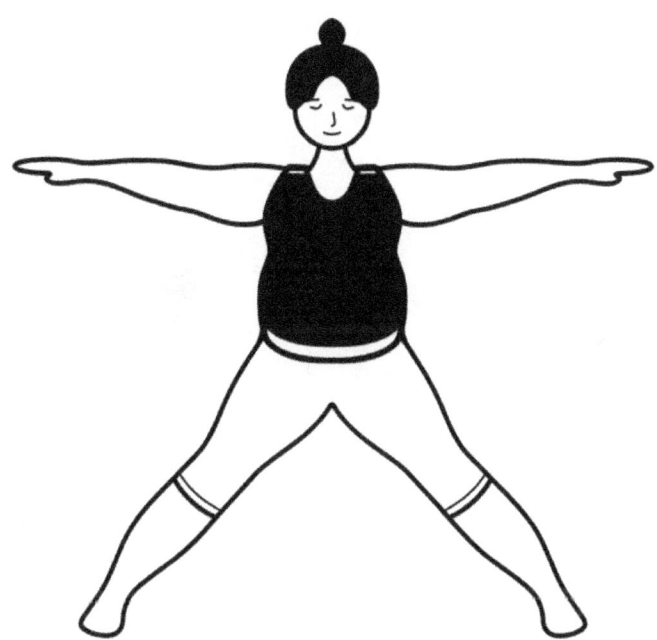

4. Press down firmly through your heels, straighten your legs, and engage your thighs to lift the kneecaps. Root evenly through all four corners of both feet.
5. Stand in your strength. Breathe deeply here for 4–8 rounds, letting your body feel expansive, steady, and alive.

SUPPORTED BRIDGE POSE
Setu Bandha Sarvangasana

1. Lie on your back with your knees bent and the soles of your feet flat on the floor, about hip-width apart.
2. Extend your arms along the floor, reaching your fingertips toward your heels. You should be able to just barely touch the backs of your heels—this helps with proper foot placement.
3. Keep your feet parallel and press down into the soles to gently lift your hips off the mat.
4. Slide a yoga block, folded blanket, or a sturdy book under your sacrum (the flat, bony area at the base of your spine). Let your pelvis rest securely on the support.

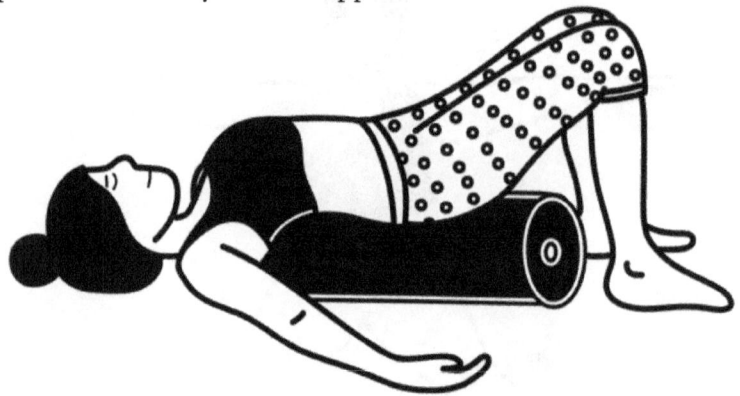

5. Keep your arms resting alongside your body, palms up or down—whatever feels best. Close your eyes. Soften your jaw. Let your breath settle into your belly.
6. Stay here for several minutes if it feels good, letting your body melt into the stretch. This is a passive backbend, so there should be no strain. If you feel any discomfort in your lower back, gently remove the support and come down.
7. To release, press into your feet to lift your hips slightly, slide the support out, and then slowly lower your spine back to the mat, one vertebra at a time.

TABLE TOP   Bharmanasana

1. Come down to the floor on your hands and knees. Align your knees under your hips, with your feet pointing straight back behind you. Place your palms directly under your shoulders, fingers spread wide and pointing forward.
2. Gaze down softly between your hands and flatten your back, creating one long, neutral line from your tailbone to the crown of your head.
3. Press into your palms to gently lift through the arms, drawing your shoulders away from your ears. Engage your belly by hugging your navel slightly in toward your spine.

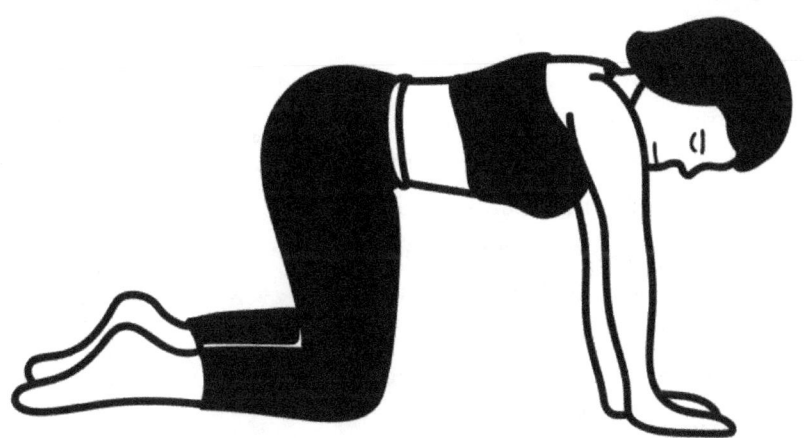

4. Extend your tailbone back and your crown forward to lengthen your spine in both directions.
5. Breathe deeply and hold for 1–3 full breath cycles.

Note:

Use this pose as a foundational shape for movement or to ground yourself in stillness.

TREE POSE   Vrksasana

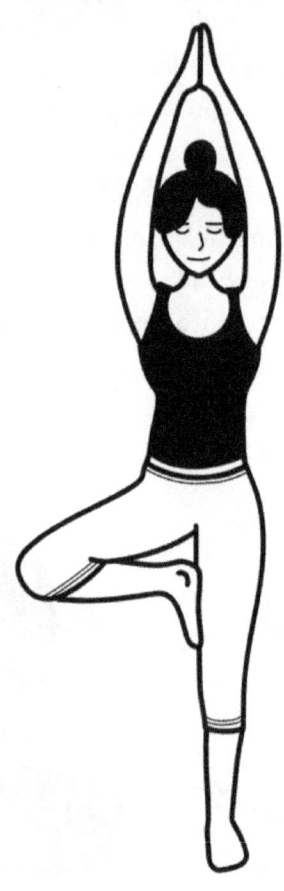

1. Begin in Mountain Pose (Tadasana). Spread your toes and press your feet firmly into the mat. Create a soft micro-bend in your knees to avoid locking them. Tilt your pelvis down slightly, drawing your front hip points toward your lower ribs to gently engage your lower belly.
2. Inhale deeply to lift through your chest, and exhale as you slide your shoulder blades down your back. Find a steady gazing point in front of you—something that won't move. This is your drishti.
3. Place your hands on your hips and lift your right foot, placing it either on your left inner thigh, calf, or ankle—wherever feels stable for you today. *Avoid pressing directly on the knee joint.*
4. Press your foot and standing leg into one another—equally, gently—finding stability through mutual resistance. Square your hips toward the front and level out your pelvis.
5. When you feel steady, bring your hands together at your heart center in prayer, or reach your arms overhead like branches growing toward the sun.
6. Hold for several slow, steady breaths, then return to Mountain Pose with control. Repeat on the other side.

TWO KNEE SPINAL TWIST
Jaṭhara Parivartanāsana

1. Begin lying on your back with your knees bent and feet flat on the floor. Lift your feet, keeping the knees and feet together, and draw your thighs up so your knees are stacked over your hips at a 90-degree angle.
2. Open your arms wide into a T-shape, palms facing up. Exhale slowly as you lower both knees to the left, keeping your shoulders grounded and your knees at hip height.
3. Encourage your right shoulder to soften toward the ground, allowing gravity to guide your twist. Gaze can be up or gently toward the right fingertips, depending on your neck comfort. Hold here for at least three deep rounds of breath.

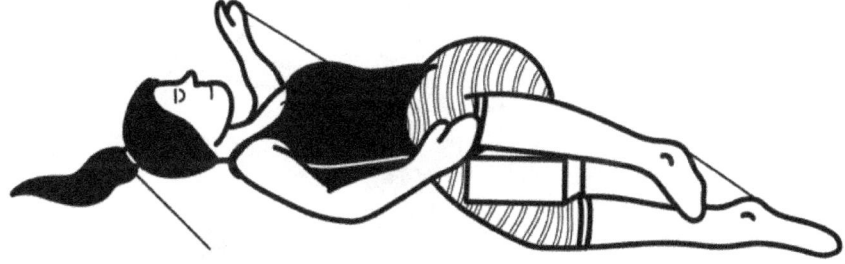

4. To come out of the pose, press your palms into the floor and engage your abdominal muscles. Inhale to lift your knees back to center, bringing them over your chest.
5. Hug your knees with both hands. On your next exhale, draw your thighs into your chest and gently lift your head and chest toward your knees. Keep your shoulders grounded as your head lifts.
6. Lower your head and shoulders back to the mat. Take a few breaths, then repeat on the other side, dropping the knees to the right and softening the left shoulder down.

WARRIOR II — Virabhadrasana II

1. Face the long edge of your mat, coming into a wide stance with your feet parallel and your arms extended straight out from your shoulders. Your ankles should be approximately beneath your wrists.
2. Turn your right foot and knee to face the front of the mat. Let your left toes turn slightly in toward the upper left corner. Bend your right knee and stack it directly over your right ankle.
3. Ground down evenly through both feet. Press into the outer edge of your back foot and feel your legs strong and rooted. Keep the crown of your head stacked over your pelvis, and your shoulders aligned over your hips.

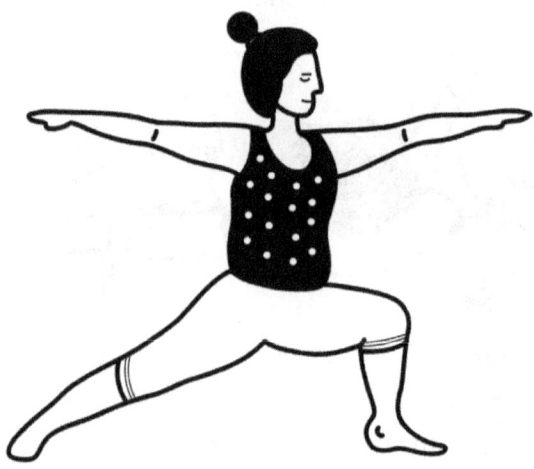

4. Reach actively through both arms—forward and back—and turn your head to gaze past your right fingertips. Settle into the strength of the pose. Hold for 5 to 10 breaths.
5. To come out, exhale and press firmly through your feet. Inhale to straighten your front leg and return your feet to parallel, facing the long edge of the mat.
6. Repeat on the other side, stepping into the strength of the pose with presence and grace.

Yoga Quick Guide

This quick-reference guide highlights key yoga poses from the chapter, their primary benefits, and suggested uses. Use it as a supportive tool to reconnect with your body, breath, and nervous system.

Yoga Pose	Primary Benefit / Use
Airplane Pose	Improves balance; strengthens legs and core
Banana Pose	Stretches the side body; relieves tension along the spine
Bird Dog	Enhances core stability and spinal alignment
Cat/Cow, Seated	Mobilizes the spine; increases seated flexibility
Cat/Cow	Warms up spine; syncs breath and movement
Chair Pose, Twisted	Strengthens legs; improves balance and digestion
Chair Pose	Builds heat; strengthens thighs and stamina
Child's Pose	Grounds; soothes the nervous system
Cobra Pose	Strengthens the spine; opens the chest
Downward Facing Dog	Full-body stretch and reset
Fetal Pose	Promotes rest and gentle spinal alignment
Folded Butterfly Pose	Opens hips and inner thighs; calms the nervous system
Forward Fold	Lengthens hamstrings; calms the mind

Seated Forward Bend	Stretches spine; calms nervous system; promotes introspection
Forward Fold, Wide-Legged	Opens hamstrings and inner thighs; releases spinal tension
Garland Pose	Opens hips; supports digestion; grounds the body
Goddess Pose	Strengthens legs and pelvic floor; awakens inner feminine energy
Half Camel Pose	Gently opens chest and spine; builds flexibility
Half Bow Pose	Opens chest and shoulders; improves posture
Half Frog Pose	Stretches thighs, groin, and abdomen
Half Lord of the Fishes	Stimulates digestion; increases spinal mobility
Half Pigeon Pose	Opens hips; releases stored tension
Halfway Lift	Lengthens spine; improves posture awareness
Happy Baby	Opens hips; relieves lower back tension
High Plank	Builds core and shoulder strength
Hero Pose	Stretches thighs and ankles; promotes stillness and grounding
Horizon's Lunge	Opens hips and side body; improves balance
Knees to Chest	Stretches lower back; massages abdominal organs

The Yoga Postures

Legs Up the Wall Pose	Relieves fatigue; calms the nervous system
Lizard Pose	Deeply opens hips; enhances flexibility
Locust Pose	Strengthens back and legs; supports posture
Mountain Pose	Grounds and centers; promotes awareness
Puppy Pose	Opens shoulders and spine; calms the mind
Rabbit Pose	Stretches spine and neck; soothes nervous system
Reclined Bound Angle	Opens hips and chest; enhances circulation
Reclining Eagle Twist	Releases spinal tension; opens shoulders and hips
Reclined Figure 4 Pose	Stretches glutes and hips; improves mobility
Runner's Lunge	Strengthens legs; opens hips and chest
Seated Staff Pose	Strengthens spine; prepares body for forward bends
Seated Forward Fold	Stretches back body; calms mind
Seated Sun Salutations	Warms up body with breath-linked movement
Seated Torso Circles	Mobilizes spine; awakens core and fluidity
Seated Twist	Aids digestion; increases spinal flexibility

Sphinx Pose	Gentle heart-opener; builds spinal awareness
Star Pose	Builds balance and presence; energizes the body
Supported Bridge Pose	Opens chest and hips; gently strengthens the spine
Table Top	Foundational neutral position; supports warm-ups
Tree Pose	Improves balance and focus; strengthens legs
Twisted Chair	Builds strength and detoxifies; improves spinal mobility
Two Knee Spinal Twist	Releases lower back tension; calms the nervous system
Warrior II	Builds strength, stamina, and focus

Moving Forward, In Your Body

You've just explored a powerful library of yoga postures—each one chosen to help you reconnect with strength, stillness, and sensation.

But these aren't just shapes on a mat.

They're invitations back into your body. Back into presence. Back into feeling.

Whether you're following your healing plan or simply moving through what feels good today, let your body lead. Some days will ask for rest. Others, for movement. Both are valid. Both are medicine.

To keep this practice alive:
- Return often. Let the poses meet you where you are.

- Sync movement with breath. Let each inhale and exhale guide you home.
- Stay curious. This is not about perfection—it's about presence.
- Use support. Props, pauses, and modifications are part of the work.

Whatever brought you here—pain, curiosity, or the desire to feel more—this space is yours.

Your body is not the barrier.

Your body is the way through.

The Meditation Practices

Your mind is not the enemy—it's just overwhelmed.
In stillness, you give it space to soften. To listen. To return.

Meditation isn't about emptying your thoughts—it's about tending to them gently.

Through repetition, rhythm, and breath, you come home—not just to calm, but to clarity.

Not just to silence, but to self.

Sit With Yourself

The Power of Sacred Words

Language holds lineage. Every Sanskrit word you'll encounter in this section is a thread—connecting you to ancient roots, deep wisdom, and the essence of healing. These mantras weren't chosen for tradition alone. They were selected for resonance. Whether spoken aloud or whispered silently, mantra meditation helps regulate your nervous system, ground your attention, and reshape old internal narratives.

In this section, you'll find simple meditations using Sanskrit mantras—each paired with emotional or sexual challenges explored in this book. Choose the one named in your healing plan, or let your intuition guide you. Repeat it slowly for 3–5 minutes. Let it steady your breath. Let it settle your system. Let it shift you.

Mantras That Move You

Emotional Resonance, Meaning, and What to Expect

Each mantra below supports a distinct emotional or energetic pattern. You won't need them all—just the one aligned with your healing plan. Let it be your anchor.

Mantra	Meaning	Emotional Tone	What to Expect
Satya	Truth	Grounding, authenticity, clarity	A sense of rootedness and alignment with your inner truth. Helpful when confusion, fear, or overthinking dominate.
Aham	I am	Self-worth, identity, connection	A stronger sense of self and belonging. Reconnects you to your inherent value and personal truth.
Swaha	Surrender	Release, openness, letting go	Relief from internal pressure and control. Helps dissolve shame, soften resistance, and create space for new patterns.

Healing Mantra Map

Each concern listed here is paired with a Sanskrit mantra that speaks directly to its emotional or energetic roots. These aren't just sounds. They're statements. Let it guide your breath, shape your attention, and return you to presence.

Concern / Barrier	Mantra (Sanskrit)	Why This Mantra
Hypoactive Sexual Desire	Satya (truth)	Reclaims your inner truth—what you want, what you feel, and what you deserve.

Sexual Arousal Disorder	Aham (I am)	Restores connection to presence and self-worth—'I am here, I am alive, I can feel.'
Sexual Aversion Disorder	Satya (truth)	Dismantles internalized shame and invites you to meet your story with honesty and care.
Hypersexuality	Aham (I am)	Brings you back to your center. Helps you discern your needs from your coping strategies.
Anorgasmia	Swaha (surrender)	Gently releases control and expectation—allowing space for sensation and pleasure to unfold.
Vaginismus	Swaha (surrender)	Softens where the body braces. Supports letting go of unconscious tension and fear.
Dyspareunia	Swaha (surrender)	Invites ease and trust. Helps dissolve patterns of guarding or holding around pain.
Vaginal Atrophy	Swaha (surrender)	Encourages healing and acceptance during a time of physical transition and change.
Vulvodynia	Swaha (surrender)	Soothes chronic tension and supports emotional release tied to persistent pain.

Endometriosis	Swaha (surrender)	Helps metabolize pain and grief while inviting tenderness toward the pelvic space.
Low Self-Esteem	Aham (I am)	Affirms your inherent worth and identity—grounding you in who you are beyond your struggles.
Poor Body Image	Satya (truth)	Challenges distorted beliefs by calling in the deeper truth of your body's value and beauty.
Self-Love Challenges	Aham (I am)	Reminds you of your wholeness. Builds inner connection through steady, loving repetition.
Unrecognized Trauma	Satya (truth)	Creates space to name what has been hidden. A gentle call to witness and reclaim your story.

You'll find the full breakdown of each mantra practice in the pages ahead.

Mantra Meditation: Satya

Best For: Hypoactive Sexual Desire Disorder (HSDD), Poor Body Image (PBI), Sexual Aversion Disorder (SAvD), Unrecognized Trauma (UT)

Overview

Satya means "truth." This mantra is a quiet return to what is real—for you, in this moment. It invites you to meet yourself with honesty and presence. After breath and movement, *Satya* helps clear space for your truth to rise—without judgment, without force. It's not about arriving at an answer. It's about being willing to listen.

How to Practice

1. Find a comfortable, supported seat. Let your body feel held.
2. Gently close your eyes and take a few grounding breaths.
3. Begin repeating the word *Satya* silently in your mind.
4. Let the rhythm be soft, steady. Don't force it.
5. When thoughts come, notice them—and gently return to your mantra.
6. Continue for 3–5 minutes. When you feel complete, let the mantra fade and slowly open your eyes.

A Note to Remember

The mind will wander. That's not a problem—it's part of the practice. Your mantra is simply the path you return to, again and again. No perfection. Just presence.

Mantra Meditation: Aham

Best For: Hypersexuality, Low Self-Esteem, Self-Love Challenges, Sexual Arousal Disorder

Overview

"Aham" means *I am*—a mantra of identity, worth, and presence. Used after breathwork and movement, it helps center you in the quiet truth of your being. You're not trying to get anywhere—you're returning to what's already here. Aham invites you to settle into yourself without judgment or effort.

How to Practice:

1. Sit in a comfortable, upright position. Let your hands rest naturally.
2. Close your eyes. Take 3–5 steady breaths to ground.
3. Begin silently repeating the mantra *aham* in your mind.
4. If your thoughts wander, gently come back to the mantra without criticism.
5. Continue for 3–5 minutes, letting your body soften and your breath flow naturally.
6. When complete, pause in stillness before you open your eyes.

Remember:

You don't need to fight your thoughts. Just let them pass—like weather moving through the sky. Your mantra is the stillness beneath it all.

Mantra Meditation: Swaha

Best For: Anorgasmia, Dyspareunia, Endometriosis, Vaginal Atrophy, Vaginismus, Vulvodynia

Overview

Swaha means *surrender*. This mantra invites you to soften—into sensation, into stillness, into the parts of yourself that don't need to try so hard. After breath and movement, *Swaha* becomes a gentle release valve for tension, expectation, and performance. It's not about doing—it's about letting go.

How to Practice:

1. Find a comfortable seated position. Let your body feel supported.
2. Close your eyes and take a few quiet breaths to settle in.
3. Begin silently repeating the mantra *swaha* in your mind.
4. When thoughts arise, let them pass. Come back to the mantra without force.
5. Continue for 3–5 minutes, allowing the sound to soften you from within.
6. When complete, pause before opening your eyes and returning to the day.

Remember:

You're not failing when your mind wanders. You're practicing when you return.

When You're Ready to Return

This chapter isn't one you'll read just once.

It's meant to be returned to.

Use what you need.

Skip what you don't.

Come back whenever your mind or body asks for something more.

Let this be your quiet guide.

Your rhythm.

Your return.

Chapter 15

The Mindset Map

Journaling, Cognitive Shifts, and the Story You're Rewriting

This chapter is designed to be used every time you engage with your Healing Plan.

When the somatic work brings you back into your body, this is where you meet what rises.

Here, you'll reflect, reframe, and reconnect—with the thoughts, beliefs, and meanings that shape your experience of sex, self, and safety.

This chapter includes:

- Daily journaling prompts to support integration of breath, movement, and meditation practices
- Cognitive reframing tools to identify, challenge, and shift limiting or unhelpful thought patterns
- Affirmations to reinforce adaptive neural pathways rooted in self-trust and embodied truth

This isn't about forcing positivity. It's about meeting your mind with compassion.

Naming what hurts.

Rewriting what no longer serves.

And practicing the beliefs you're ready to grow into.

The Journaling Practices

Your body has spoken. Your breath has opened. Your awareness has softened.

Now, it's time to listen with your pen.

Journaling is where everything you've felt, moved through, and breathed into begins to land.

It's not just reflection—it's revelation. A space where your inner world becomes visible.

Not to judge. Not to fix. But to witness.

The Page is a Portal

In this section, you'll write as a way of honoring what's rising.
You'll meet the thoughts, sensations, and stories that shape your experience—and begin to gently reshape them.

This chapter is divided into three sections, each supporting a different layer of your healing:

1. **Daily Reflections (Post-Practice)** – Body-based prompts to use right after movement, breathwork, or mantra. These help you reconnect to sensation, shift awareness into your body, and track subtle changes over time.
2. **Reframing Limiting Thoughts (CBT-based)** – Belief-focused prompts to explore inherited stories, shift self-talk, and rewrite the inner narratives around sex and self-worth.
3. **Affirmations to Rewire and Reclaim** – Short, potent truths to speak, write, or hold in your awareness. They support neural rewiring and emotional realignment.

You don't have to do it perfectly. You don't have to do it every day. But when you put pen to page, something powerful happens:

You open a portal.

Section 1. Daily Reflections (Post-Practice)

These questions are meant to be explored right after your movement, breath, and meditation practice. They help you tune in to where sensation lives in your body, how it shifts, and what your physical responses might be trying to tell you.

Think of these as gentle check-ins with your inner world. You're not trying to "solve" anything—just to witness, feel, and record what arises.

Some prompts focus on physical sensation. Others explore energy or emotion. All of them invite insight—not performance.

This isn't journaling for writing's sake. It's journaling for remembering. For reconnecting with your embodied experience in real time.

Buy yourself a beautiful journal—the kind that feels good in your hands—and copy these questions into its first pages. Return to them often. Let your journal become a mirror, a record, a quiet place to come home to.

After each practice session, take a quiet moment with yourself. Each condition explored in this book includes a few body-based prompts tailored to your unique healing path. These aren't abstract—they're grounded in your lived, physical reality: what your body felt, noticed, or wanted.

You'll return to this page often. Let it be a soft landing place. A place to listen inward.

These prompts are not a checklist, and you don't need "right" answers—only honest ones. You also won't need to do all of them. I've selected the most relevant prompts for your specific sexual wellness concern and placed them in a quick-reference table on the next page. You'll also see your recommended journaling focus clearly outlined in your Healing Plan. No guesswork—just guidance.

Let this be a daily ritual of remembrance. A way to stay in relationship with the parts of you that are awakening.

Where to Begin: Body-Centered Journal Prompts by Sexual Health Concern

Hypoactive Sexual Desire Disorder	What sensations are present in the lower half of your body while in Puppy Pose? Where does your awareness naturally drift? How does your body want to move in this pose? Side to side? Up and down? Back and forth?
Sexual Arousal Disorder	Where do you feel energy flowing while in cobra pose? After the pose, where do those sensations linger? As you pressed your pelvis into the mat, what did you notice in your body's response?
Sexual Aversion Disorder	Where do you feel your power while in Goddess Pose? With your hips and chest open, your thighs strong, and your spine lengthened–where in your body do you notice tension? Where do you feel warmth or aliveness rising?
Hypersexuality / Compulsive Sexual Behavior	Throughout your flow or during a particular pose, when did you feel the most in control of your full self? As you hold Chair Pose with strength in your thighs, hips, and core– where do you feel the most tension building? Where in your body do you feel the most in control?

Anorgasmia	As you moved into Half Bow Pose, where does energy concentrate in your body? Does your energy flow to a specific part of your body when you are in your half-bow pose? Does your body respond more to the buildup of heat—or the sensation of release when you let go?
Dyspareunia	As you stretch your groin, inner thighs, and hips in your reclined bound angle pose, where do you feel the most release in your body? When your legs were up the wall, what feelings came through your body? What shifted?
Vaginismus	Where did your attention go in your body when you pressed your hips forward & up into bridge pose? What feelings washed over you when your legs were up the wall?
Vaginal Atrophy	Where does the heat build most in your body while in your garland pose/squat? What part of your body feels the most powerful right now after completing your practice?
Vulvodynia	As your hips press forward in lizard pose, did you notice your breath slow or quicken? Where in your body did you notice the most sensation—comfort or discomfort?
Endometriosis	What feelings come up in your body while you performed your seated torso circles? How does concentrating on compression feel in your abdomen?

Low Self-Esteem	In Warrior II, where in your body do you feel your personal power rising from? How does your body's energy shift from Warrior II to Star Pose? Which pose makes you feel most connected to yourself–and why?
Poor Body Image	What movement or pose makes you feel the most connected to yourself? How does your body want to move in the most intuitive way? What feels the best?
Self-Love	What happens in your body as you make space in your throat while in your half camel pose? In the full expression of your camel pose, where do you feel the most sensation?
Unrecognized Trauma	Does folding forward or opening up feel better in your body? What pose made you feel the most grounded? What pose made you feel the safest in your body?

You've reflected on what your body is telling you—now it's time to explore what your thoughts are saying. Let's move into the next section: reframing limiting beliefs.

Section 2. Reframing Limiting Thoughts

Using CBT to Challenge the Narratives That Hold You Back

This section invites you to explore the stories and beliefs that shape your experience of sex, pleasure, and self-image. Rooted in Cognitive Behavioral Therapy (CBT), these prompts help you notice outdated scripts, reframe limiting thoughts, and make space for new truths to emerge.

You don't need to do this every day. In fact, once or twice a week is enough to create meaningful change—and your Healing Plan will highlight the specific prompt most relevant to your current process. Use this section when something tender rises to the surface, or anytime you feel ready to meet yourself more honestly.

How to Use This Section

These reflections are different from your daily movement or breath practices. They're deeper dives into your mental and emotional patterns—best done slowly, gently, and with lots of self-compassion.

What to expect:

- Some prompts will lead to instant insight.
- Others might unfold gradually, with realizations appearing days later.
- You may feel resistance—that's normal. Stay curious.

Let this be a space of gentle exploration. You're not here to "fix" yourself. You're here to witness your thoughts, question what's no longer true, and reshape your inner narrative with care.

What You'll Practice

In this section, you'll be invited to:
- Identify limiting beliefs you've been carrying
- Explore where they came from (family, trauma, culture, past partners)
- Ask new, liberating questions
- Reframe old thoughts using real-life evidence or self-compassion

These exercises are based in Cognitive Behavioral Therapy (CBT), a powerful, evidence-backed method that starts with one truth:

Thoughts are not facts.

The Journaling Practices

Many of our thoughts are skewed—shaped by assumptions, expectations, fears, judgments, or inherited stories. In CBT, we call these cognitive distortions or thinking traps. The good news? You can learn to recognize them, interrupt them, and shift them toward something more accurate and supportive.

What It Looks Like

Step 1: Identify and Reframe

We start by challenging a single limiting belief. You'll name the thought, ask key questions, and reframe it with compassion and clarity.

Example

Limiting Thought: *"I shouldn't need as much rest as I do."*

Questions to Ask:

- Should my need for rest always stay the same?
- Isn't rest essential to health and vitality?
- Couldn't rest be a form of wisdom, not weakness?

Reframed Thought: "My rest needs are allowed to shift based on my body, my life, and my choice."

Now try your own. Use the template below to complete 1–3 of your own reframes in your journal each week:

Reframing Template:

- Limiting Thought:
- Questions to Ask:
- Reframed Thought:

Step 2: Be Curious

These journaling prompts are not about getting it "right"—they're about getting real.

Let them be a place to return to, reshape, and rewrite as often as you need.

Some weeks you'll go deep. Other times, just a few words. That's enough.

Pick a few to explore each week—or move freely between them. There's no perfect pace, only your process.

Over time, you're not just answering questions. You're rewriting the narrative.

Body Beliefs

- What do I currently believe about my body?
- Where did those beliefs come from?
- How have they shaped my self-image or intimacy?
- How do these beliefs show up in the bedroom or when I'm emotionally vulnerable?
- Do I feel deserving of pleasure, rest, or being seen—just as I am?
- How do these beliefs affect the way I receive touch, compliments, or desire?

Sexual Beliefs

- What do I believe about sex or sexuality?
- Where did those beliefs originate?
- How have they shaped my experiences, struggles, or desires?
- How do these beliefs impact how I communicate what I want (or don't want)?
- Do I feel pressure to perform, please, or hide parts of myself?
- How do these beliefs influence the kind of connection I seek—or avoid?

Step 3: Reframe the Loop

Each week, as you reflect on your body and sexual beliefs, certain thoughts will rise to the surface.

Some will be loud and obvious. Others will hum quietly beneath the surface.

This is where you meet them.

These are the mental loops—the old stories that keep you stuck in shame, disconnection, or self-doubt.

They may sound like:

"I'm too much." "I'm not enough." "I should be over this by now."

But they're not the truth. They're rehearsed. This practice helps you name those thoughts and gently reshape them.

Not with force. With attention.

You're not just rewriting a sentence—you're repairing your relationship to your body, your worth, and your desire.

Now try your own. Reframe the loop related to body or sexual beliefs.
- What thought do I most want to reframe right now?
- Limiting Thought:
- Reframed Thought:

Repeat this process for up to two more thoughts if you'd like.

Step 4: Reframes Around Pleasure

This step is about clearing the internal blocks that stand between you and joy.
- What brings me genuine pleasure and bliss—solo or partnered?
- What thoughts, beliefs, or fears block me from accessing more of it?

- What would I need to ask for, believe, or let go of to fully receive that pleasure?

Pleasure isn't just about the moment—it's about the life that holds it.

Once you've explored what you need, want, and deserve…

It's time to dream bigger.

Step 5: Write the Life You Long For

If you could be the author of your dream life…

- What would that life look like if nothing held you back?
- How would you feel in it—physically, emotionally, spiritually? Think BIG.
- How would it feel in your body? In your relationships?
- What beliefs would you need to release to step into that vision?

Write without limits. Let your longing lead.

Do it once. Or a million times. As many as it takes.

You Did Something Brave

By stepping into this space—by questioning old beliefs, exploring your desires, and imagining a life beyond your limits—you've done something courageous.

This isn't about perfection. It's about presence.

Some days will bring clarity. Other days, you'll simply show up. Both matter. Both create change.

Over time, this inner work reshapes your thoughts, softens shame, and lays the foundation for deeper connection, confidence, and sexual wellness.

Let this be your reminder:

You are not broken.

You are becoming.

Section 3: Affirmations to Rewire and Reclaim

Words shape worlds—especially the ones we speak to ourselves.

After you've listened to your body and explored your thoughts, affirmations offer a chance to speak directly into your healing. These aren't just feel-good phrases. They're intentional declarations—designed to soften old beliefs, soothe your nervous system, and anchor you in truth.

Each affirmation is paired with a concern or barrier you may be working through. You don't have to believe it fully right away. Let it land softly. Say it aloud. Whisper it in the mirror. Write it down. Repeat it as often as needed.

Let this be your closing ritual—a moment of self-compassion and clarity.

Your List of Affirmations to Choose From

These affirmations are here to inspire, not confine.

Let them serve as a starting point—a spark. If something resonates, claim it. If something doesn't, change it. And if your soul offers you a phrase that's not written here, write it down and make it yours.

You are your own authority when it comes to healing and reclaiming your body, your voice, and your pleasure.

Safety & Self-Worth
- I am enough just the way I am.
- My body is a good body.
- I am kind.
- I am thoughtful.
- I am trustworthy.
- I am exactly where I need to be.
- I validate myself first before seeking validation from others.
- I deserve to love myself.
- I believe in myself.
- I believe in the power of my love for myself.

Pleasure & Body Connection
- I desire to feel good in my body.
- I deserve to feel good in my body.
- My body deserves pleasure right here, right now.
- I don't need to change in order to feel pleasure.
- I'm learning to pleasure my own body.
- I'm learning to prioritize my pleasure.
- I touch my body lovingly.
- I'm proud of my body.
- My body is powerful.
- I am full of sexual energy.
- I deserve to reach orgasm.

Awareness & Mind-Body Trust
- I intuitively know what my body wants.
- I listen to what my body is telling me.
- I tune in to my own needs and wants.
- I sit with discomfort, not pain.
- I learn when to push and when to pause.
- I trust when to push and when to pause.
- I challenge my thoughts when my mind wants sex but my body is scared.

Consent, Control & Communication
- I am in control of my headspace.
- I speak my truth.
- I share my truth with those I trust.
- I communicate my needs to my loved ones.
- I talk openly with my partner about my desires.
- I talk openly with my partner when I'm not in the mood.
- I define what intimacy is for me.
- I am not a mind-reader.

- My partner can't read my mind.
- Sex is something I participate in, not something that is done to me.

Sexual Identity & Desire
- I am a sexual being.
- Sex is more than intercourse.
- Sex is more than penetration.
- Sex is connection.
- Sex is not everything to me.
- I want to feel aroused.
- I want to feel sexual.
- I'm curious about my sexuality.
- I want to have blissful sex.
- I want to orgasm.
- I want to climax.
- I don't need an orgasm to feel fulfilled sexually.

Giving & Receiving Love
- I am open and willing to receive pleasure.
- I am open and willing to give myself pleasure.
- I give love.
- I receive love.
- I deserve to be my #1.
- I am my first priority.
- I take care of myself willingly.
- I am sexy.
- I am desired.
- I am cared for.
- I share my sexual interests and erotic curiosities.
- I surround myself with people I can trust.
- I live my life without fear.
- I speak my truth without fear.

The Journaling Practices

After you choose the affirmations that resonate most, consider adding one more—an anchor that directly supports the healing journey you're on.

Below are specific affirmations aligned with each of the healing paths in this book. These are offered as gentle companions, helping you speak into the exact space where you're growing. Let them guide your focus. Let them remind you that your body—and your healing—deserve tenderness.

Affirmations for Each Healing Plan

1. **Reigniting Desire – Hypoactive Sexual Desire Disorder**
   "I deserve to feel good in my body."

2. **Waking the Spark Within – Sexual Arousal Disorder**
   "I intuitively know what my body wants."

3. **Replacing Fear with Freedom – Sexual Aversion Disorder**
   "I'm curious about my sexuality."

4. **Reclaiming Control, Rebuilding Trust – Hypersexuality / Compulsive Sexual Behavior**
   "I believe in the power of my love for myself."

5. **The Rise Toward Release – Anorgasmia**
   "I am open and willing to receive pleasure."

6. **Making Space for Pleasure – Dyspareunia**
   "I'm learning to prioritize my pleasure."

7. **Unwinding the Body's No – Vaginismus**
   "My body is powerful."

8. **Reclaiming Radiance – Vaginal Atrophy**
   "My body deserves pleasure right here, right now."

9. **Soothing the Fire, Restoring Your Voice – Vulvodynia**
   "I listen to what my body is telling me."

10. **Listening to the Body's Truth – Endometriosis**
    "I sit with discomfort, not pain."

11. **Becoming the Mirror You Trust – Low Self-Esteem**
"I am in control of my headspace."

12. **Rewriting the Body's Birth Story – Poor Body Image**
"My body is a good body."

13. **Loving Yourself Like You Mean It – Self-Love Barrier**
"I deserve to love myself."

14. **Healing What Wasn't Heard – Unrecognized Trauma**
"I speak my truth without fear."

The End of the Map, The Start of the Path

Your words carry power.

Every time you speak life over your body, your mind listens. Every time you declare truth over your experience, your nervous system softens. This isn't about pretending everything is perfect. It's about choosing a different conversation—one rooted in possibility, in presence, in self-trust.

Over the last two chapters, you've been invited into deeper awareness.

You've begun to reflect on your breath. You've started to notice your body in new ways. You've considered what's been unspoken. You've let truth rise—even if only quietly, inside yourself.

These practices may seem simple—but they're anything but small. They are rewiring the foundation from which you relate to your body, your pleasure, your power.

So—keep going.

Return to these tools whenever you need to remember.

Add to them. Rewrite them. Let them evolve as you do.

Let them become a conversation between the version of you who's healing… and the version of you who's already whole.

Because now, you're ready.

What comes next is the heart of this book:

a healing plan made just for you.

Chapter 16

Healing Plans for the 14 Core Concerns

Now it's time to bring it all together.

In this section, you'll find individualized healing plans for each of the 14 sexual wellness concerns covered in this book. These are not rigid protocols. They're structured, supportive frameworks designed to help you move forward—one day at a time.

You are not meant to do all 14.

Based on your self-assessment—or an existing diagnosis—you've likely identified one or more concerns that resonate with your experience. Start there.

Each plan follows the same daily structure, in this order:

1. Breathwork
2. Movement
3. Meditation
4. Journaling/CBT
5. Affirmations

Each day takes about 27–30 minutes to complete.

The *Movement* section of each plan is written as a flow-style sequence—guiding you from one posture into the next, like a gentle choreography for your body. If you'd like support getting into each pose, flip back to the Yoga Postures in chapter 14 starting on page 133. You'll find step-by-step instructions and illustrations there to help you move with confidence and care.

Reading through the movement sequences may feel overwhelming at first—especially if your body isn't used to being guided this way. That's okay. These cues are meant to spark felt experience. Let your body take the lead. Over time, the instructions will start to make more sense—not just in your head, but in your muscles, breath, and rhythm. Let it feel awkward until it becomes embodied.

If you're working with more than one concern, alternate the healing plans throughout the week.

For example:
- Plan A: Sundays, Tuesdays, Thursdays
- Plan B: Mondays, Wednesdays, Fridays
- Saturday: repeat, mix and match, or rest

This work is meant to be sustainable. Go at your own pace.

What matters most is that you continue to show up.

The Healing Plans

Reigniting Desire – Hypoactive Sexual Desire Disorder

Waking the Spark Within – Sexual Arousal Disorder

Replacing Fear with Freedom – Sexual Aversion Disorder

Reclaiming Control, Rebuilding Trust – Hypersexuality / Compulsive Sexual Behavior

The Rise Toward Release – Anorgasmia

Making Space for Pleasure – Dyspareunia

Unwinding the Body's No – Vaginismus

Reclaiming Radiance – Vaginal Atrophy

Soothing the Fire, Restoring Your Voice – Vulvodynia

Listening to the Body's Truth – Endometriosis

Becoming the Mirror You Trust – Low Self-Esteem

Rewriting the Body's Birth Story – Poor Body Image

Loving Yourself Like You Mean It – Self-Love Block / Barrier

Healing What Wasn't Heard – Unrecognized Trauma

Reigniting Desire – Hypoactive Sexual Desire Disorder

Breathwork (5 min):	Yoga Pose Flow (10 min):	What Hypoactive Sexual Desire Disorder Looks Like
Breath of Fire Page: <u>109</u>	1 Seated Cat/Cow 2 Child's Pose 3 Table Top 4 Traditional Cat/Cow 5 Puppy Pose 6 Down Dog 7 High Plank	A persistent lack of interest in sex, often causing frustration or confusion. The person may love their partner but feel no desire for intimacy, leading to relationship strain. This is not due to another medical condition, stress, or medication.

Movement:

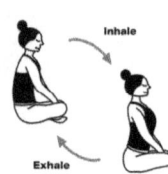

Start in a comfortable seat. Hands on knees. Begin with **Seated Cat/Cow** movements. Inhale, press your heart forward, proud chest, as you drag your hands back towards your hips. Exhale. Round your back for cat pose by bringing your hands back to your knees.

Use your inhale to move your body forward and your exhale to move back. Repeat 3 times.

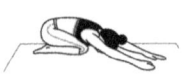

Come into **Child's pose**. You can bring your big toes together, knees wide. Reach your hands forward. Take 3 breaths here. Slowly reach towards your right keeping your hips planted towards your heels. Take 5 breaths. Come back through center and reach to your left. Take 5 breaths.

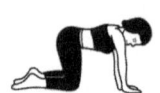

Come back to center. Lift your body into **Table Top**. Put your hands under your shoulders, knees under hips. Look back at your feet and make sure you can't see them. Inhale.

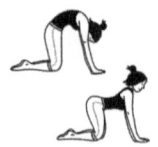

Exhale, dome your back for **Cat pose**. Inhale into your **Cow pose**. Belly will drop and your chest will lift. Exhale. Round your spine, bring your gaze in between knees. Using your breath, add in big barrel rolls. Big circular motions to your right and big circular motions to your left. Repeat 5 times.

Healing Plans for the 14 Core Concerns

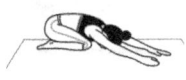 Sink back down into **Child's pose**. Slowly walk your hands forward and allow your bottom to lift up. Find a comfortable place for your chin (on the floor or put your forehead to the earth). Allow your heart to melt down as your hips are lifting up. Breathe deep, filling your lungs and releasing.

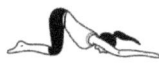 Wiggle your bottom while it's high in the air. **Puppy pose**. Take 5 deep, sensual breaths here. Connect to yourself.

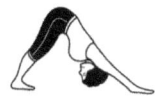 When you release, come into **Downward-facing Dog**.

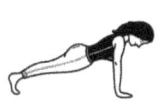 Lift your heels (you're on your toes). Shift your gaze to your belly button. As you do this, dome your upper back like cat pose.

Keep your body moving, gently drift your body forward into a **High Plank**, letting your belly sink down and your knees may drop. Your shoulders are stacked over your wrists and your heels above your toes. Lift back up, bend your knees to a hover.

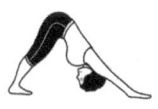 Scoop your booty back towards your heels as you round back into **Downward-facing Dog**. You're creating a wave-like motion here—flow with your breath as you move. Repeat this three times.

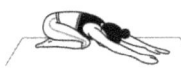 Sink back down into **Child's pose** for 5 breaths. Sit back into your seated pose.

Reigniting Desire – Hypoactive Sexual Desire Disorder

Meditation (5 min):

Satya (Truth)

Page 203

Repeat your mantra silently for 3–5 minutes, letting it anchor your awareness. If thoughts come, gently return to the mantra.

Remember: Thinking is only natural. Notice what arises—don't give it your attention.

Body-Based Reflections (5 min):

Use these prompts immediately after movement and meditation to stay connected to your body:

1. What sensations are present in the lower half of your body while in Puppy Pose? Where does your awareness naturally drift?

2. How does your body want to move in this pose? Side to side? Up and down? Back and forth?

Reframe Limiting Thoughts (CBT) (5 min):

What came up for you today?

Refer back to pages: 213-218

- Limiting thought:

  _____

- Questions to ask:

  _____

- Reframed thought:

  _____

Healing Plans for the 14 Core Concerns

> **Be Curious...**
>
> Here are examples for your writing reflection, but feel free to pick your own.
>
> - Do I feel deserving of pleasure, rest, or being seen—just as I am?
> - Do I feel pressure to perform, please, or hide parts of myself?
> - How do these beliefs influence the kind of connection I seek—or avoid?

> **Affirmation to Anchor the Practice**
>
> *I deserve to feel good in my body.*
>
> Repeat this affirmation silently or aloud as you close your practice. If it doesn't feel fully true yet—don't worry. Let it become a seed you're planting.

> *"When you give your thoughts space to stretch and your body space to feel, healing starts to speak."*

Waking the Spark Within – Sexual Arousal Disorder

Breathwork (5 min):	Yoga Pose Flow (10 min):	What Sexual Arousal Disorder Looks Like
Lion's Breath Page 110	1 Half Lord of the Fishes 2 Table Top 3 Bird Dog Pose 4 Half Frog Pose 5 Sphinx 6 Cobra 7 Child's Pose 8 Rabbit's Pose	The body does not respond to sexual stimulation as expected. A person may want to feel aroused but struggles with a lack of physical response, like no lubrication or genital sensitivity, even in situations that should be exciting.

Movement:

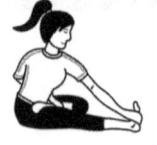

Start in a comfortable seat. Extend your left leg in front of you and take your right foot and cross it over your left leg. The outside edge of your right foot is flush with the outside of your left thigh. Plant your right hand behind you, so your right elbow is straight.

Hook your left elbow outside of your right knee and inhale lengthen your spine, exhale twist to your right. **Half Lord of the Fishes pose**. Breathe here.

Untangle your legs. Prepare for the opposite side. Release your right leg, extend it down. Bend your left knee, place the outside, side edge of your left foot outside of your thigh. Extend your left arm behind you, so it is straight. Hook your elbow so it's attached to your left knee. Inhale for length, exhale twist to your left. Breathe here.

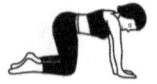

Come back to your center, release your leg and move into your **Table Top**.

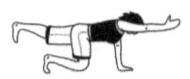

Extend your right leg behind you (you're on your toe) with weight on your left leg. Lift your left arm in front of you (off the earth, in line with your shoulder).

Lift your right leg off the earth. Take a big breath in for length and as you exhale, connect your left elbow to your right knee, so you're crunching in towards your belly. Inhale open and exhale crunch. **Bird Dog pose**. Repeat 3 times at your own pace.

Release your knee to the earth. Extend left leg behind you as you reach your right arm forward. Lift both limbs off the earth, inhale for length, exhale crunch your elbow to your left knee— pull your energy in. Repeat on the left side for 3 rounds.

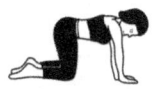

Return back to **Table Top**. Lower down to your belly. Bring your arms to a goal post, so elbows are bent. Inhale here, then a slow exhale.

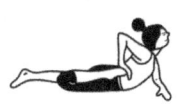

Slowly drag your right knee towards your right elbow into **Half Frog**. Release your left cheek to the earth. 5 breaths here.

Extend your right leg. Slowly bend your left knee, so it reaches toward your left elbow. Turn your head. Rest your right cheek on the earth. Take 5 breaths.

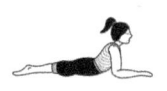

Lower your leg back down to the earth. Lift your heart—your forearms are on the earth, elbows under shoulders. Palms face down. Gently pull your belly off the ground. Hold for 3 seconds. **Sphinx pose**. Release your belly back down. Repeat this three times, remembering to lift your heart as you pull your belly off the earth.

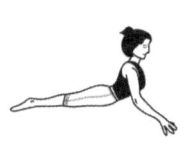

Lower all the way down. Bring forehead to the earth and make sure you are on the tops of your feet. Press the tops of your feet down. Bring your hands to your sides, thumbs in line with your nipples. Gently press your hands into the earth.

Press tops of feet down as you lift your heart off the earth and into **Cobra pose**. Hold for 3 breaths. 3 slow and deliberate inhales and exhales. Slowly release down. Pause.

Come right back into it, as your heart lifts from the earth. Find a fluid motion by leading with your chin and pulling body weight down and rolling your body right back up into cobra pose on inhale. Lead with your chin, ground down. Repeat this fluid motion 5 times.

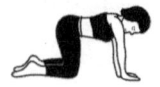
Lift your body back into **Table Top**. Bring your big toes to touch.

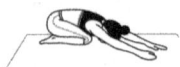
Reach your arms forward into **Child's pose**. Hold for five breaths.

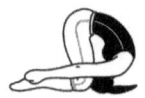
Gently take your hands, reach them around your body so they connect to your heels as you press your body weight forward onto the crown of your head, if it will allow—pull all your energy inward towards your center. **Rabbit pose**. Hold for 5 to 8 breaths.

Gently release down. Slowly lift your body on an inhale and come to an easy seated position.

Waking the Spark Within – Sexual Arousal Disorder

Meditation (5 min):

Aham (I am)
Page 204

Repeat your mantra silently for 3–5 minutes, letting it anchor your awareness. If thoughts come, gently return to the mantra.

Remember: Thinking is only natural. Notice what arises—don't give it your attention.

Body-Based Reflections (5 min):

Use these prompts immediately after movement and meditation to stay connected to your body:

1. Where do you feel energy flowing while in cobra pose? After the pose, where do those sensations linger?
2. As you pressed your pelvis into the mat, what did you notice in your body's response?

Reframe Limiting Thoughts (CBT) (5 min):

What came up for you today?
Refer back to pages: 213-218

- Limiting thought:
  _____

- Questions to ask:
  _____

- Reframed thought:
  _____

> **Be Curious...**
>
> Here are examples for your writing reflection, but feel free to pick your own.
>
> - What do I currently believe about my body?
> - Where did those beliefs come from?
> - How have they shaped my self-image or intimacy?

> **Affirmation to Anchor the Practice**
>
> *I intuitively know what my body wants.*
>
> Repeat this affirmation silently or aloud as you close your practice. If it doesn't feel fully true yet—don't worry. Let it become a seed you're planting.

> *"When you give your thoughts space to stretch and your body space to feel, healing starts to speak."*

Replacing Fear with Freedom – Sexual Aversion Disorder

Breathwork (5 min):	Yoga Pose Flow (10 min):	What Sexual Aversion Disorder Looks Like
Box Breathing Page 112	1 Child's Pose 2 Table Top 3 Down Dog Pose 4 Mountain Pose 5 Wide-legged Forward Fold 6 Star Pose 7 Goddess Pose	Intense fear, disgust, or avoidance of sexual activity. Even the thought of intimacy may cause anxiety, panic, or distress. This can be due to past trauma or negative experiences, but not always.

Movement:

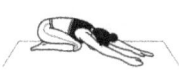

From your comfortable seat, come down into **Child's pose** with big toes together and knees wide. Reach your hands through towards your feet, connect your hands to your heels. Take 5 breaths.

Keep your lower body in child's pose as you lift up, place your right hand behind your right foot. Push hips forward as you reach left arm to the sky, angling yourself back.

Gently release down, take your left hand, place it behind your left foot. Push hips forward as you reach your right arm up and behind you to reach towards the back of the room. Bring your hips back down. Repeat from side to side 3 times.

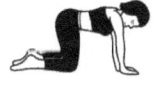

Come into **Table Top** with hands under shoulders and knees under hips. Look back; make sure your feet are not visible. Rock side to side. Inhale to left, exhale to right, 3 breath cycles.

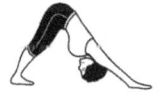

Flip your toes, lift your hips to get into **Downward-facing Dog**. Pedal your feet. Lift heels, take slow steps forward; round your back. Bend knees as you get closer to the mat.

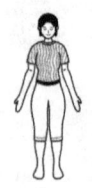

When you're at the top, slowly roll up to stand, one vertebra at a time. Drop your shoulders. Arms by your sides, palms facing out. **Mountain pose**. Take 5 breaths.

Turn to left or right, facing the long edge of your mat. Lift whatever leg brings you down the mat.

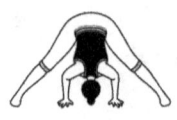

Take a big step into a wide-legged stance. With knees slightly bent and arms out to your sides parallel to the floor, hinge at your hips until you feel a gentle tug in all directions. **Wide-legged Forward Fold**. Take 3 breaths.

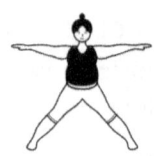

Slowly roll back up to stand, keeping legs wide. Reach both arms wide and up to the sky. **Star pose**. Inhale, look to the sky, Exhale, bring head to center for 3 breaths.

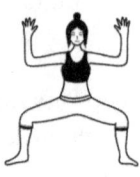

Adjust feet so heels point in and toes point out. Bend knees and elbows into **Goddess pose**. Your arms will look like a goal post. Inhale. Lift arms, straighten legs. Exhale, bend knees. Bend elbows, goddess pose. Repeat 5 times, linking breath to movement.

Toe heel your feet back together, and shake it out, whatever feels good. Then find a comfortable seat.

Replacing Fear with Freedom – Sexual Aversion Disorder

Meditation (5 min):

Satya (Truth)

Page 203

Remember: Thinking is only natural. Notice what arises—don't give it your attention.

Body-Based Reflections (5 min):

Use these prompts immediately after movement and meditation to stay connected to your body:

1. Where do you feel your power while in Goddess Pose?

2. With your hips open, your thighs strong, and your spine lengthened–where in your body do you notice tension? Where do you feel warmth or aliveness rising?

Reframe Limiting Thoughts (CBT) (5 min):

What came up for you today?

Refer back to pages: 213-218

- Limiting thought:

  _____

- Questions to ask:

  _____

- Reframed thought:

  _____

> **Be Curious...**
>
> Here are examples for your writing reflection, but feel free to pick your own.
>
> - What do I believe about sex or sexuality?
> - Where did those beliefs originate?
> - How have they shaped my experiences, struggles, or desires?

> **Affirmation to Anchor the Practice**
>
> *I'm curious about my sexuality.*
>
> Repeat this affirmation silently or aloud as you close your practice.
>
> If it doesn't feel fully true yet—don't worry. Let it become a seed you're planting.

"When you give your thoughts space to stretch and your body space to feel, healing starts to speak."

Healing Plans for the 14 Core Concerns

Reclaiming Control, Rebuilding Trust – Hypersex/Comp Sexual Behavior

Breathwork (5 min):	Yoga Pose Flow (10 min):	What Hypersexuality / Compulsive Sexual Behavior Looks Like
Alternate Nostril Breathing Page 113	1 Seated Twist 2 Table Top 3 Down Dog 4 Mountain Pose 5 Chair Pose 6 Twisted Chair 7 Forward Fold 8 Child Pose	Frequent, intense sexual urges or behaviors that feel out of control. Even when acting on them, the person does not feel satisfied. It can interfere with relationships, work, and daily life.

Movement:

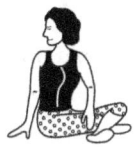

Start in your comfortable seat. Bring your palms together. Feel your thumb knuckles come together, touching your sternum. Big breath in as you gently twist to your right keeping hands at heart center. Press into sternum, breathe in. Exhale, twist deeper—**Seated Twist**.

Inhale, slowly come back to center, release your hands. As you exhale, move from your hips and fold your body down as far as you can go with arms on the earth. Gently lift your body back up. Place hands back at heart center. Inhale.

On your exhale, twist to the left. Keep thumb knuckles attached to your sternum. Inhale, twist a little deeper. Slowly come back to center, fold your body weight forward. Inhale. Exhale.

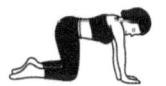

Come into **Table Top**. Shoulders are above your hands and knees below hips. Take a moment to reset with 3 cycles of breath.

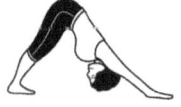

Flip your toes. Lift your hips into **Down Dog**. Pause here. Breathe. When you're ready, lift your heels and take slow steps forward to the front of your mat.

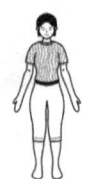
Bend your knees a lot and slowly rise, 1 vertebra at a time into **Mountain pose**. Feet firmly planted, slight bend in the knees. Lift your shoulders up towards your ears, roll your shoulder blades back and down, palms forward. Stand tall and feel strong in mountain pose.

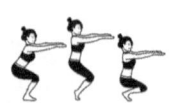
Inhale, lift your arms to the sky—as you exhale, bend your knees to come into **Chair pose**. Arms reaching forward. Feel that your bottom is reaching behind you. Lift your hands to your heart, rest them there with palms touching and thumbs pressing together.

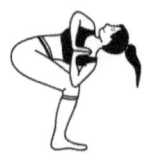
Keep this connection as you take a big breath in and twist to your right, keeping your hands connected to your sternum. Take three breaths in your **Twisted Chair pose**.

Come back to center. Release your hands, and on an exhale, Forward Fold. Inhale and lift back into chair pose. Connect hands to your heart. Inhale. As you exhale, twist to your left.

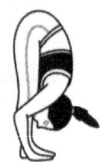
Connect to your center. Take 3 breaths in your chair pose twist. Release your hands as you fold forward once again. Dangle them for 3 breaths. On your inhale, slowly lift to stand and reach arms to the sky. As you exhale, release arms down. Fold.

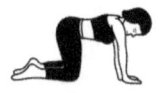
When you're ready, crouch down and gently bring your knees to the earth. Find your way back into **Table Top**. Breathe.

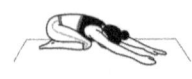
Grab your pillow. Bring your big toes together, knees will be as wide as your mat. Place the pillow underneath your heart and come into a supported **Child's pose**. Stay here for 5-8 breath cycles.

When ready, gently lift back up into your easy seat.

Reclaiming Control, Rebuilding Trust – Hypersex/Comp Sexual Behavior

Meditation (5 min):

Aham (I am)
Page <u>204</u>

Repeat your mantra silently for 3–5 minutes, letting it anchor your awareness. If thoughts come, gently return to the mantra.
Remember: Thinking is only natural. Notice what arises—don't give it your attention.

Body-Based Reflections (5 min):

Use these prompts immediately after movement and meditation to stay connected to your body:

1. Where in your body do you feel the most in control?
2. As you hold Chair Pose with strength in your thighs, hips and core–where do you feel tension building?

Reframe Limiting Thoughts (CBT)

What came up for you today?

Refer back to pages: <u>213-218</u>

- Limiting thought:

  _____

- Questions to ask:

  _____

- Reframed thought:

  _____

> **Be Curious…**

Here are examples for your writing reflection, but feel free to pick your own.

- Do I feel pressure to perform, please, or hide parts of myself?
- How do these beliefs influence the kind of connection I seek—or avoid?

> **Affirmation to Anchor the Practice**
>
> *I believe in the power of my love for myself.*
>
> Repeat this affirmation silently or aloud as you close your practice. If it doesn't feel fully true yet—don't worry. Let it become a seed you're planting.

> *"When you give your thoughts space to stretch and your body space to feel, healing starts to speak."*

Healing Plans for the 14 Core Concerns

The Rise Toward Release – Anorgasmia

Breathwork (5 min):	Yoga Pose Flow (10 min):	What Anorgasmia Looks Like
Breath of Joy Page 114	1 Mountain Pose 2 Airplane Pose 3 Table Top 4 Half Bow 5 Child Pose	Difficulty or inability to reach orgasm despite sufficient stimulation. This can happen in all situations or only in specific ones, leading to frustration and distress.

Movement:

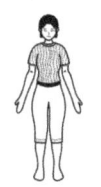

Stand in your **Mountain pose**. Feel your feet grounded in the earth.

Inhale. Bring your right knee to your chest, grab and squeeze your knee in towards your body. Create a micro bend in your left knee for balance. Hold for 3 breaths.

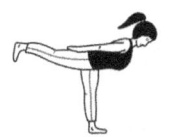

Gently kick your right leg behind you and allow it to float as you move your arms to your sides. Keep your arms lifted, palms facing down. Feel your chest lift. **Airplane pose**. 3 breaths here.

If you need a stable support, like a counter top, it's OK (ignore arm movements while floating your leg back). Gently bring your knee back to your chest. Hold. Adjust your left leg if you need to stay balanced. Find momentum and release back into your airplane pose.

Repeat this movement 3 times, shifting from knee bent and lifted at chest to kicking back with legs and reaching back with arms for airplane pose.

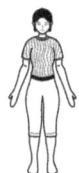

When your finished, return your right leg to the ground and come back into **Mountain pose**. Stand tall. Chest proud. Inhale. Exhale.

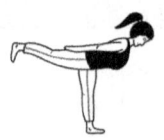 Inhale, grab your left knee. Repeat the same motions you just did, but on the opposite side. You're coming in and out of **Airplane pose** (knee to chest and gently kicking it back) for 3 rounds.

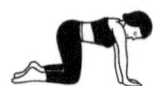 Bring your body down into **Table Top**. Give yourself a moment to sway your hips back and forth. Arrive here.

When you're ready, slowly lower all the way down onto your belly. Extend your arms out into a T or into a goal post and gently roll onto your right hip. You should feel sensation in your right pectoral muscle.

You can lift your left leg and place your left foot behind you with a bent knee for more. Hold for 8 breaths.

Roll onto your belly, reset with a breath. Slowly roll onto left hip and repeat on this side. Hold for 8 breaths. Come back down to your belly. Pause.

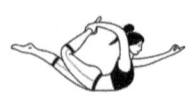 Bend your right knee and reach your right hand around to the outside of the right foot, either grabbing your ankle or your foot, whichever is more comfortable for you. Extend your left arm forward with palm facing the earth.

Press your right foot into your hand as you lift your right side. If you feel like you want more, lift your left arm off your mat and your left leg will lift off the earth. Hold for 5 breaths. **Half Bow**, right side. Release all the way down.

Bend your left knee and reach your left hand around to the outside of the left foot, either grabbing your ankle or your foot. Extend your right arm forward with palm facing the earth. Press your left foot into your hand as you lift your left side.

If you feel like you want more, lift left arm off mat and left leg will lift off the earth. Hold for 5 breaths. **Half Bow**, left side.

Release all the way down.

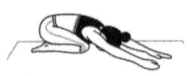 Come into **Child's pose**, hold for 5 breaths.

Find your easy seat.

Healing Plans for the 14 Core Concerns

The Rise Toward Release – Anorgasmia

Meditation (5 min):

Swaha (Surrender)
Page 205

Repeat your mantra silently for 3–5 minutes, letting it anchor your awareness. If thoughts come, gently return to the mantra.
Remember: Thinking is only natural. Notice what arises—don't give it your attention.

Body-Based Reflections (5 min):

Use these prompts immediately after movement and meditation to stay connected to your body:

1. As you move into Half Bow Pose, where does energy concentrate in your body?
2. Does your body respond more to the buildup of heat—or the sensation of release when you let go?

Reframe Limiting Thoughts (CBT) (5 min):

What came up for you today?

Refer back to pages: 213-218

- Limiting thought:

  _____

- Questions to ask:

  _____

- Reframed thought:

  _____

> **Be Curious...**

Use these reflection prompts weekly (or when you're ready for deeper insight):

- Where am I limiting my thoughts?
- What are your beliefs about your body? Where did those beliefs come from?
- What do I want to reframe most?
- What gives me the most sexual pleasure and bliss?

    Solo sex/masturbation: _____

    Partnered experiences: _____

- What do you need to reframe or ask for in order to experience more pleasure?

> **Affirmation to Anchor the Practice**
>
> *I am open and willing to receive pleasure.*
>
> Repeat this affirmation silently or aloud as you close your practice. If it doesn't feel fully true yet—don't worry. Let it become a seed you're planting.

> *"When you give your thoughts space to stretch and your body space to feel, healing starts to speak."*

Healing Plans for the 14 Core Concerns

Making Space for Pleasure – Dyspareunia

Breathwork (5 min):

Abdominal Breathing
Page 116

Yoga Pose Flow (10 min):

1 Knees to Chest
2 Two Knee Spinal Twist
3 Reclined Bound Angle
4 Banana Pose

Props: 2 pillows, blanket, timer

What Dyspareunia Looks Like

Persistent pain during intercourse or any type of penetration. This pain can be sharp, burning, or deep, making intimacy uncomfortable or even impossible.

Movement:

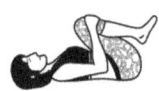

Come to lay down on your back. Take a moment to wiggle around and get comfortably flat. Adjust your shoulder blades, adjust your bottom. When you're ready, pull both of your knees into your chest. This is your pose—**Knees to Chest**. Hold for 5 slow breaths.

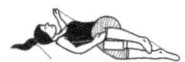

Release both of your knees to your right as you extend your arms out like a T. Feel your left shoulder touch the earth. Use your pillows to prop in between your knees for comfort. **Two Knee Spinal Twist** to the right. Hold here for 2 minutes.

Hug your knees into your chest. Reset with a breath in and out. Again. In and out. Release both knees to your left, propping a pillow or two in between. Extend both of your arms out like a T. Feel your right shoulder touch the earth. **Two Knee Spinal Twist** to the left. Hold for 2 minutes.

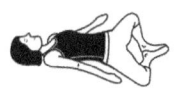

Pull both of your knees into your chest. Grab both of your pillows, place 1 on the right and 1 on the left. Feel the soles of feet come together as knees splay open wide, resting on each pillow. Place your right hand on your chest and your left hand on your belly.

Supported **Reclined Bound Angle**. Hold for 2 minutes.

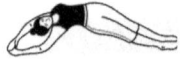 Bring both of your hands to the outsides of your knees, pull them in together. Extend your legs long down the mat. Keep hips at center as you reach your legs down and to the right. Your arms will lift above your head and reach up and to your right. You will be in the shape of a banana. **Banana pose** to the right. Hold for 2 minutes.

Come back to center. Bring your legs to the left. Lift your arms above your head and reach to the left. **Banana pose** to left. Hold for 2 minutes. Come back to center.

When ready, find a comfortable seat.

Healing Plans for the 14 Core Concerns

Making Space for Pleasure – Dyspareunia

Meditation (5 min):

Swaha (Surrender)
Page 205

Repeat your mantra silently for 3–5 minutes, letting it anchor your awareness. If thoughts come, gently return to the mantra.
Remember: Thinking is only natural. Notice what arises—don't give it your attention.

Body-Based Reflections (5 min):

Use these prompts immediately after movement and meditation to stay connected to your body:

1. As you stretch your groin, inner thighs and hips in your reclined bound angle pose, where do you feel the most release in your body?
2. When your legs were up the wall, what feelings came through your body?

Reframe Limiting Thoughts (CBT) (5 min):

What came up for you today?

Refer back to pages: 213-218

- Limiting thought:

　_____

- Questions to ask:

　_____

- Reframed thought:

　_____

> **Be Curious...**
>
> Here are examples for your writing reflection, but feel free to pick your own.
>
> - Do I feel deserving of pleasure, rest, or being seen—just as I am?
> - How do these beliefs affect the way I receive touch, compliments, or desire?

> **Affirmation to Anchor the Practice**
>
> *I'm learning to prioritize my pleasure.*
>
> Repeat this affirmation silently or aloud as you close your practice. If it doesn't feel fully true yet—don't worry. Let it become a seed you're planting.

> *"When you give your thoughts space to stretch and your body space to feel, healing starts to speak."*

Unwinding the Body's No – Vaginismus

Breathwork (5 min):
Cooling Breath
Page 118

Yoga Pose Flow (10 min):
1 Table Top
2 Cat/Cow
3 Happy Baby
4 Supported Bridge Pose
5 Legs Up the Wall

Props: 2 pillows, blanket, timer

What Vaginismus Looks Like
The muscles around the vaginal opening involuntarily tighten, making penetration painful or impossible. This can happen even when the person wants to engage in intimacy.

Movement:

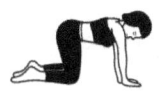

From your comfortable seat. Transition onto your hands and knees into **Table Top pose**. Take a moment to set yourself up. Wiggle where you need to. Lift one hand, circle the wrist and set it back down. Lift the opposite hand, circle the wrist and set it back down.

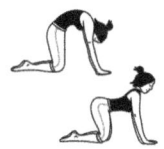

Prepare for your **Cat/Cow** movements. Stack your shoulders over your wrists and make sure your knees are stacked under your hips. Inhale. Lift your chin, drop your belly. Exhale, round your spine and shift your gaze in between your knees. Repeat this 5 times with your breath and a focus on moving from your belly button. Be slow and deliberate. Feel your way through.

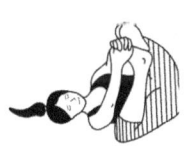

Find your way onto your back as you hug your knees into your chest. Find your peace fingers and wrap them around your big toes, or grasp outside of your feet as you anchor into your low back. Draw your elbows towards hips. **Happy Baby pose**. Find a playful movement side to side or make figure eights with your low back. Don't be shy. Really move here. Play in this pose for 2 minutes.

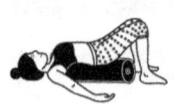
Find stillness. Drag your knees into your chest, release your feet to earth. Grab a pillow or your prop, press your feet into the earth as you lift your hips. Place your pillows or prop under your low back. Make sure your shoulders are touching the earth and your bottom is lifted at an incline. **Supported Bridge pose**. Hold this pose for 3 minutes.

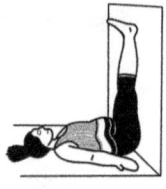
Move close to a flat wall. Draw your right knee into your chest. Pause. Draw your left knee into chest. Pause for 2 breaths. Scoot your bottom towards the wall (no need to touch wall, but you can, if you want to). Extend your right leg to the sky, then extend your left leg to the sky. Allow both legs to be fully supported by the wall. Your arms are either at your sides or reaching to your feet. Shoulders melt into the earth. **Legs Up the Wall**. Hold this pose for 2 minutes. Or longer if you have the time.

Slowly release both legs back to the earth. Remove your pillow. Drape body into fetal posture on either side and pause here.

Lift yourself up to a comfortable seat.

Healing Plans for the 14 Core Concerns

Unwinding the Body's No – Vaginismus

Meditation (5 min):

Swaha (Surrender)
Page 205

Repeat your mantra silently for 3–5 minutes, letting it anchor your awareness. If thoughts come, gently return to the mantra.
Remember: Thinking is only natural. Notice what arises—don't give it your attention.

Body-Based Reflections (5 min):

Use these prompts immediately after movement and meditation to stay connected to your body:

1. Where did your attention go in your body when you pressed your hips forward & up into bridge pose?
2. What feelings washed over you when your legs were up the wall?

Reframe Limiting Thoughts (CBT) (5 min):

What came up for you today?
Refer back to pages: 213-218

- Limiting thought:

  _____

- Questions to ask:

  _____

- Reframed thought:

  _____

> **Be Curious...**
>
> Here are examples for your writing reflection, but feel free to pick your own.
>
> - What do I currently believe about my body?
> - Where did those beliefs come from?
> - How have they shaped my self-image or intimacy?

> **Affirmation to Anchor the Practice**
>
> *My body is powerful.*
>
> Repeat this affirmation silently or aloud as you close your practice. If it doesn't feel fully true yet—don't worry. Let it become a seed you're planting.

> *"When you give your thoughts space to stretch and your body space to feel, healing starts to speak."*

Healing Plans for the 14 Core Concerns

Reclaiming Radiance – Vaginal Atrophy

Breathwork (5 min):	Yoga Pose Flow (10 min):	What Vaginal Atrophy Looks Like
Three-Part Breath Page 124	1 Reclining Eagle Twist 2 Mountain Pose 3 Garland Pose 4 Child Pose	After menopause, estrogen levels drop, leading to vaginal dryness, irritation, and discomfort during sex. This can make intimacy painful and reduce natural lubrication.

Movement:

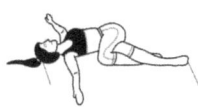

Come to lie down on your back. Pull both knees into your chest. Take a moment to breathe here. Wiggle out the tension in your lower back. When you're ready, cross your right knee over your left. You can double cross at the ankles or not. Release your legs down to the right. Arms extend to a T into your **Reclining Eagle Twist** to the right. Hold for 8 breaths.

Come back to center, untangle your legs. Cross your left knee over your right this time and drop to your left. Extend arms to a T. **Reclining Eagle Twist** to the left. Hold for 8 breaths.

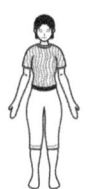

Pull your knees back into your chest. Rock and roll forward and back multiple times. Come through a seat and stand tall in your **Mountain pose**.

Inhale, reach your arms to the sky. As you exhale, draw hands to heart center. Hold for 1 round of breath. Look down at your feet and toe heel them out wide, until your toes are out and heels are in. You can have a stance as wide as your mat if that feels good.

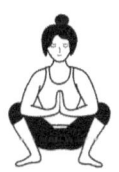

Slowly release your bottom down to the earth into **Garland pose**. Use a block beneath you for support. Hold for 5 breaths.

Inhale, come to stand. Exhale back into your squat. Use your breath to move through standing and squatting. Repeat this sweeping motion 5 times. Pay attention to your breath.

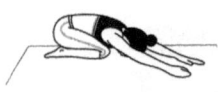When you're ready, come down to a seat. Bring your knees off to one side. Move your body anyway you need to, so you can lift onto your knees. Wiggle your bottom, and re-set here. Allow your big toes to touch and let your knees open wide. Reach yourself forward and sink down into your **Child's pose**. Feel your way into the version of this pose that feels right for you. Hold for 8 breaths. Slow. Deliberate. Check in with yourself.

Bring your knees to your side and come back to your easy seated position.

Healing Plans for the 14 Core Concerns

Reclaiming Radiance – Vaginal Atrophy

Meditation (5 min):

Swaha (Surrender)
Page 205

Repeat your mantra silently for 3–5 minutes, letting it anchor your awareness. If thoughts come, gently return to the mantra.
Remember: Thinking is only natural. Notice what arises—don't give it your attention.

Body-Based Reflections (5 min):

Use these prompts immediately after movement and meditation to stay connected to your body:

1. Where does the heat build most in your body while in your garland pose/squat?
2. What part of your body feels the most powerful right now after completing your practice?

Reframe Limiting Thoughts (CBT) (5 min):

What came up for you today?
Refer back to pages: 213-218

- Limiting thought:

  _____

- Questions to ask:

  _____

- Reframed thought:

  _____

> **Be Curious...**
>
> Here are examples for your writing reflection, but feel free to pick your own.
>
> - Do I feel pressure to perform, please, or hide parts of myself?
> - How do these beliefs influence the kind of connection I seek—or avoid?

> **Affirmation to Anchor the Practice**
>
> *My body deserves pleasure, right here, right now.*
>
> Repeat this affirmation silently or aloud as you close your practice. If it doesn't feel fully true yet—don't worry. Let it become a seed you're planting.

> *"When you give your thoughts space to stretch and your body space to feel, healing starts to speak."*

Healing Plans for the 14 Core Concerns

Soothing the Fire, Restoring Your Voice – Vulvodynia

Breathwork (5 min):

Bee Breath
Page 120

Yoga Pose Flow (10 min):

1 Two Knee Twist
2 Fetal Pose
3 Table Top
4 Lizard Pose
5 Wide-Legged Forward Fold

What Vulvodynia Looks Like

Chronic vulvar pain, burning, or irritation that happens even without an obvious cause. It can make everyday activities like sitting, wearing tight clothing, or riding a bike uncomfortable or painful.

Movement:

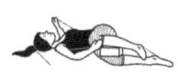

From your easy seat. Slowly come down to your back with both knees pulled into your chest. Release your knees to the right as your arms extend out like a T. Relax your top knee on your bottom knee. Use a prop if that feels good in your body. Hold here for 5 slow rounds of breath. **Two Knee Twist** to the right.

Slowly pull your knees back into your chest. Release them off to the left side. Extend your arms like a T, allow gravity to pull you down to your left. Hold for 5 breaths. **Two Knee Twist** to the left.

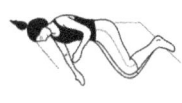

Hug both of your knees into your chest. Release to your right side for **Fetal pose**. Curl into yourself. Hold for 5 breaths. Come back to center and pull your knees in again. Rock and roll—forward and back 3 times until you land in a seat.

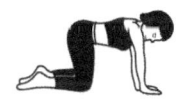

Slowly transition into **Table Top**. Get grounded here. Take a moment to check in with what you're feeling in your body. Our next pose is a lot of sensation. Prepare.

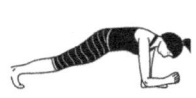

When you're ready, step your right foot outside of your right hand. Flip onto the back of your toes, shimmy your body back a little bit. Grab a prop, pillow or block and place it inside your right foot. Allow your forearms to come down to the earth. If it's too much sensation, come back onto your hands and press your hands into earth, and allow your heart to pull forward. Hold for 8 breaths. **Lizard pose**, right side.

Slowly come out of the pose and bring your left knee back in line with the right. When you're ready, slowly lift up to stand tall. You may want to pause on your knees before lifting up. Once you're standing, reset here with a natural round of breath.

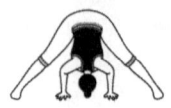

Turn your body, so you are facing the long edge of your mat. Open your legs wide, so your right foot reaches to the right corner and your left foot reaches to the left corner. Open your arms to your sides and hinge at your hips to fold forward. Eventually, your hands land to frame your head. Find a place that feels comfortable for your arms. Keep a micro-bend in the knees. **Wide-Legged Forward Fold**. Hold for 8 breaths.

Slowly cross your legs and come back to your comfortable seat.

Soothing the Fire, Restoring Your Voice – Vulvodynia

Meditation (5 min):

Satya (Truth)
Page 203

Repeat your mantra silently for 3–5 minutes, letting it anchor your awareness. If thoughts come, gently return to the mantra.
Remember: Thinking is only natural. Notice what arises—don't give it your attention.

Body-Based Reflections (5 min):

Use these prompts immediately after movement and meditation to stay connected to your body:

1. As your hips press forward in lizard pose, did you notice your breath slow or quicken?
2. Where in your body did you feel the most sensation–comfort or discomfort?

Reframe Limiting Thoughts (CBT) (5 min):

What came up for you today?
Refer back to pages: 213-218

- Limiting thought:

  _____

- Questions to ask:

  _____

- Reframed thought:

  _____

Be Curious...

Here are examples for your writing reflection, but feel free to pick your own.

- What do I currently believe about my body?
- Where did those beliefs come from?
- How have they shaped my self-image or intimacy?

Affirmation to Anchor the Practice

I listen to what my body is telling me.

Repeat this affirmation silently or aloud as you close your practice. If it doesn't feel fully true yet—don't worry. Let it become a seed you're planting.

> *"When you give your thoughts space to stretch and your body space to feel, healing starts to speak."*

Healing Plans for the 14 Core Concerns

Listening to the Body's Truth – Endometriosis

Breathwork (5 min):

4-7-8 Breathing
Page 122

Yoga Pose Flow (10 min):

1 Seated Torso Circles
2 Seated Forward Bend
3 Table Top
4 Cat/Cow
5 Down Dog
6 Half Pigeon Pose

Props: 2 pillows, blanket, timer

What Endometriosis Looks Like

Chronic pelvic pain that may worsen during menstruation, sex, or bowel movements. It's caused by tissue similar to the uterine lining growing outside the uterus. The pain can feel sharp, dull, or crampy—and it often comes with fatigue or emotional overwhelm.

Movement:

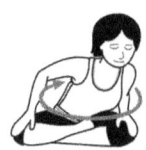

Start in a comfortable seat. Place your hands on your thighs. Sit tall. Take a big inhale, and release with a big exhale. When you're ready, make big sweeping circles with your torso to the right. Feel the movement in your spine. **Seated Torso Circles**. Repeat this motion 5 times. After the fifth, pause in the center.

Reset. Sit tall. Elongate your spine. Now move in the opposite direction. Make big sweeping circles to the left 5 times. Nice and slow. Move with intention. Pay attention to your breath. Pause for a moment here.

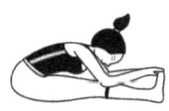

Uncross your legs, and extend both of your legs down your mat, in front of you. Grab a pillow or a block, and place it on your thighs. Slowly fold down onto the pillow, moving from your hips. Rest your head wherever it feels comfortable. **Seated Forward Bend**. Hold for 2-3 minutes.

Slowly, from the hips, come back up. Bring your right hand behind your right knee. Bring your left hand behind your left knee. Draw your knees into your chest and hold for a round of breath.

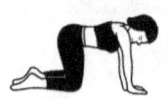
Release your knees off to the side and come through **Table Top**. Take a moment and pause here. Adjust your hands, adjust your legs. Be sure that your shoulders are stacked over wrists and knees under your hips. Inhale. Exhale. Inhale.

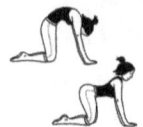
On your next exhale, play with **Cat/Cow** movements here. Inhale, lift your chin and drop your belly. Exhale, round your spine, gaze between your knees. Repeat these movements 5 times. Go slow—really feel your way through the movements.

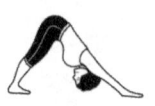
Shift your body into **Downward-facing Dog**. Pause. Adjust your stance, so you feel strong. Widen your legs, or narrow them. Whatever you need. When you're ready, extend your right leg to the sky, draw your knee to your chest 3 times.

On the last rep, slowly release your knee to the earth. Drag it towards your right wrist as you fan your right foot to the left. Be on your back toes, to control movement forward and backward.

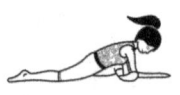
You're slowly coming down into **Half Pigeon pose**. Use a prop under your right hip. Fold your torso forward. Hold here for 3 minutes. Gently come out and extend your left leg to the sky. Pull your left knee into your chest 3 times. On the last rep, release your knee to the earth at the top of your mat—dragging it towards your left wrist. Fan your left foot to your right and pull your body weight back, so you're on top of the pose. Use your prop under your left hip. Release your heart down to the earth for **Half Pigeon pose** on the opposite side. Hold here for 3 minutes.

Slowly lift up and come back to your easy seat.

Listening to the Body's Truth – Endometriosis

Meditation (5 min):

Aham (I am)

Page 204

Repeat your mantra silently for 3–5 minutes, letting it anchor your awareness. If thoughts come, gently return to the mantra.

Remember: Thinking is only natural. Notice what arises—don't give it your attention.

Body-Based Reflections (5 min):

Use these prompts immediately after movement and meditation to stay connected to your body:

1. What feelings come up in your body while you performed your seated torso circles?
2. How does concentrating on compression feel in your abdomen?

Reframe Limiting Thoughts (CBT) (5 min):

What came up for you today?

Refer back to pages: 213-218

- Limiting thought:

  _____

- Questions to ask:

  _____

- Reframed thought:

  _____

> **Be Curious...**
>
> Here are examples for your writing reflection, but feel free to pick your own.
>
> - Do I feel pressure to perform, please, or hide parts of myself?
> - How do these beliefs influence the kind of connection I seek—or avoid?

> **Affirmation to Anchor the Practice**
>
> *I sit with discomfort, not pain.*
>
> Repeat this affirmation silently or aloud as you close your practice. If it doesn't feel fully true yet—don't worry. Let it become a seed you're planting.

> *"When you give your thoughts space to stretch and your body space to feel, healing starts to speak."*

Healing Plans for the 14 Core Concerns

Becoming the Mirror You Trust – Low Self Esteem

Breathwork (5 min):	Yoga Pose Flow (10 min):	What Low Self-Esteem Looks Like
Bellows Breathing Page 126. When you finish, check in with your physical body first: how do your cheeks feel? Your lips? Your arms? Your chest? Where do you feel the prana or energy flowing in your body? Collect that energy up and cross your arms over your chest for an embrace.	1 Mountain Pose 2 Forward Fold 3 Runner's Lunge 4 Warrior II 5 Halfway Lift 6 Star Pose	A quiet inner critic that distorts how you see yourself. You may constantly compare yourself to others, dismiss compliments, or believe you're not worthy of love, rest, or joy. It can make self-care feel like a chore instead of a birthright.

Movement:

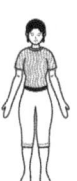

Come to stand. Find your **Mountain pose**. Release your arms, so they're down by your sides. Lift your shoulders up towards your ears and release them behind you. Drop your right ear towards your right shoulder. Part your lips and tilt the back of your head towards your spine for 3 breaths.

Come back to center. Release your left ear to your left shoulder. Keep your lips parted as you drift the back of your head towards your spine. Hold for 3 breaths.

Repeat this three times on each side.

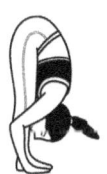

Hinge at your hips, and slowly lower all the way down, so your hands are reaching towards the earth in a **Forward Fold**.

Interlace your hands behind your knees. Bend your knees a lot as you fold down towards yourself, so your chin is reaching towards your shins. Hold here for 8 breaths.

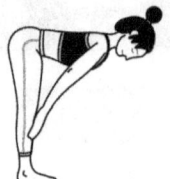

Release your hands, so they can touch the earth. Slowly lift your body halfway up with your hands on your shins. **Halfway Lift**. Exhale, bow down back into your forward fold.

Repeat this 3 times.

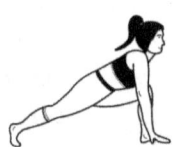

Step your right foot back into a low **Runner's Lunge**. Tent your hands to frame your front foot. Shift your gaze forward as you press your heart towards the front of your mat. Hold for 5 breaths. Lift up into a high runner's lunge.

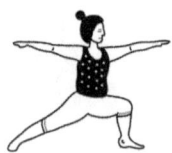

Open into **Warrior II**. Check that your back foot is parallel to the back of your mat and your front foot is at 12 o'clock. Open your wingspan, close your eyes and stay here for 8 breaths.

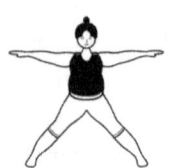

Inhale, lift both of your arms to the sky. Allow both feet to come into a stance, with your toes in, heels out, facing the long edge of your mat.

Star pose.

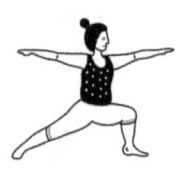

On your exhale come back to **Warrior II**. Repeat this 3 times. Moving from Warrior to Star pose.

Land in your Warrior II. Windmill your hands down to your mat.

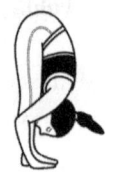

Step forward and come back into your **Forward Fold**.

Inhale, **Halfway Lift**, so your hands are on your shins.

Healing Plans for the 14 Core Concerns

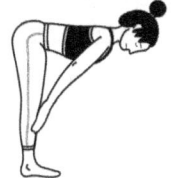

Exhale, lower down. Forward fold. Let's move to the opposite side.

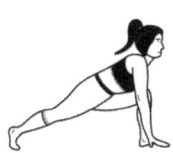

Step your left foot back into a low **Runner's Lunge**. Frame your front foot with your hands. Shine your heart forward as you press your fingertips down.

Hold this for 5 breaths. Lift into your high runner's lunge.

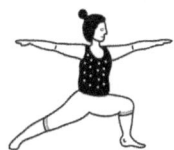

Open up into **Warrior II**. Stay here for 5 breaths.

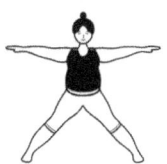

Inhale, lift both arms to the sky remembering toes in and heels out, looking towards the long edge of your mat.

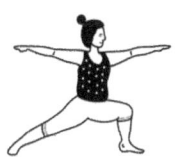

Exhale back into Warrior II. Repeat this 3 times.

Windmill your hands down to the earth.

Step forward.

Lower your knees down, and have a seat.

Becoming the Mirror You Trust – Low Self Esteem

Meditation (5 min):

Aham (I am)
Page 204

Repeat your mantra silently for 3–5 minutes, letting it anchor your awareness. If thoughts come, gently return to the mantra.
Remember: Thinking is only natural. Notice what arises—don't give it your attention.

Body-Based Reflections (5 min):

Use these prompts immediately after movement and meditation to stay connected to your body:

1. In Warrior II, where in your body do you feel your personal power rising from?
2. How does your body's energy shift from Warrior II to Star Pose?
3. Which pose makes you feel most connected to yourself–and why?

Reframe Limiting Thoughts (CBT) (5 min):

What came up for you today?

Refer back to pages: 213-218

- Limiting thought:

  _____

- Questions to ask:

  _____

- Reframed thought:

  _____

Healing Plans for the 14 Core Concerns

> **Be Curious...**
>
> Here are examples for your writing reflection, but feel free to pick your own.
>
> - What do I currently believe about my body?
> - Where did those beliefs come from?
> - How have they shaped my self-image or intimacy?
> - How do these beliefs show up in the bedroom or when I'm emotionally vulnerable?

> **Affirmation to Anchor the Practice**
>
> *I am in control of my headspace.*
>
> Repeat this affirmation silently or aloud as you close your practice. If it doesn't feel fully true yet—don't worry. Let it become a seed you're planting.

> *"When you give your thoughts space to stretch and your body space to feel, healing starts to speak."*

Rewriting the Body's Birth Story – Poor Body Image

Breathwork (5 min):	Yoga Pose Flow (10 min):	What Poor Body Image Looks Like
Equal Breathing Page 128	1 Folded Butterfly Pose 2 Table Top 3 Cat/Cow Pose 4 Child Pose 5 Down Dog 6 Runner's Lunge 7 Horizon's Lunge	Feeling numb or disconnected from your body—especially when it comes to joy, sensuality, or touch. You might struggle to notice physical cues, resist receiving pleasure, or feel like your body belongs to someone else.

Movement:

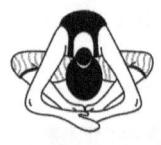

From your comfortable seat—bring the soles of your feet together and allow your knees to splay open wide. Place your hands on your feet. Inhale to open your chest. Exhale, to fold your torso down towards your feet. Feel your chin reach in towards your chest. Hold here for 8 breaths. **Folded Butterfly** pose.

Release your heart up, so it is above your hips. Pause. Bring your right hand to the outside of your right knee as you also place your left hand to the outside of your left knee. Draw both knees in together. Bring them off to one of your sides.

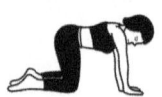

Come into **Table Top pose**. Make sure your hands are under your shoulders and your knees are under your hips. Wiggle your bottom and then find stillness for a natural round of breath.

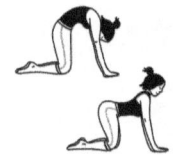

Inhale, drop your belly, lift your gaze into **Cow pose**. Exhale round your spine, shift your gaze to in between your knees for **Cat pose**. Repeat 3 times moving fluidly between cat and cow.

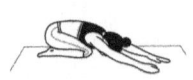

When you're done, bring your big toes together, open your knees wide.

Sink back into **Child's pose**, hold here for 5 breaths.

Healing Plans for the 14 Core Concerns

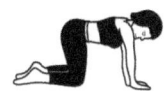
Lift back into your **Table Top**. Pause. Get aligned.

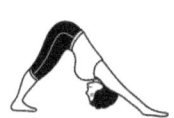
Flip your toes, lift your hips and release to **Downward-facing Dog**. Feel into your body here by finding intuitive movement—bending your knees, rolling your spine, feeling into your body.

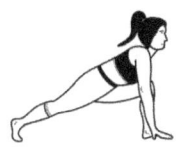
Step your right foot forward in between your hands into a low **Runner's Lunge**. Keep your hands on the earth.

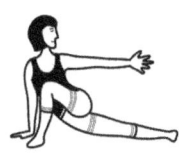
Use toe then heel movements of your right foot to bring it to your right side, landing halfway down your mat. Feel that your whole foot is on the earth. Make sure the outside of your left foot touches your mat—you'll be on the outside edge of your left foot.

Horizon's Lunge. Inhale, reach your right arm to the sky. Make a rainbow shape, reaching towards the front of your mat. Exhale, drop your hips and release your right arm down towards the earth. Repeat this motion 3 times with your breath.

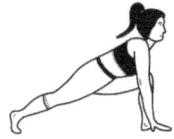
Slowly come back into your **Runner's Lunge**.

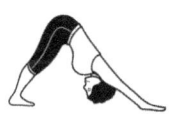
Step back into your **Downward-facing Dog**. Breathe here. Prepare for the other side.

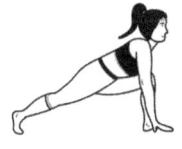
Now step your left foot forward into your **Runner's Lunge**. Toe heel your left foot to your left, landing halfway down the mat. Come to the outside edge of your right foot.

Horizon's Lunge.

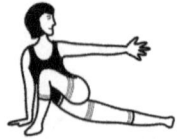

Lift your hips as you lift your left arm to the sky. Reach for the front of your mat, making a rainbow shape once again. Exhale, drop your hips, release your left hand down.

Repeat this 3 times, allowing the movement to be fluid. Breathing into it.

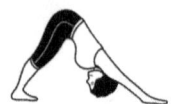

Come back into **Downward-facing Dog**.

Breathe.

Release your knees to your mat and come into an easy seat.

Rewriting the Body's Birth Story – Poor Body Image

Meditation (5 min):

Satya (Truth)
Page <u>203</u>

Repeat your mantra silently for 3–5 minutes, letting it anchor your awareness. If thoughts come, gently return to the mantra.
Remember: Thinking is only natural. Notice what arises—don't give it your attention.

Body-Based Reflections (5 min):

Use these prompts immediately after movement and meditation to stay connected to your body:

1. What movement of pose makes you feel the most connected to yourself?

2. How does your body want to move in the most intuitive way? What feels the best?

Reframe Limiting Thoughts (CBT) (5 min):

What came up for you today?

Refer back to pages: <u>213-218</u>

- Limiting thought:

  _____

- Questions to ask:

  _____

- Reframed thought:

  _____

> **Be Curious...**
>
> Here are examples for your writing reflection, but feel free to pick your own.
>
> - What do I currently believe about my body?
> - Where did those beliefs come from?
> - How have they shaped my self-image or intimacy?
> - How do these beliefs show up in the bedroom or when I'm emotionally vulnerable?
> - Do I feel deserving of pleasure, rest, or being seen—just as I am?
> - How do these beliefs affect the way I receive touch, compliments, or desire?

> **Affirmation to Anchor the Practice**
>
> *My body is a good body.*
>
> Repeat this affirmation silently or aloud as you close your practice. If it doesn't feel fully true yet—don't worry. Let it become a seed you're planting.

"When you give your thoughts space to stretch and your body space to feel, healing starts to speak."

Healing Plans for the 14 Core Concerns

Loving Yourself Like You Mean It – Self-Love Block / Barrier

Breathwork (5 min):	Yoga Pose Flow (10 min):	What Self-Love Block Looks Like:
Lion's Breath Page 110	1 Hero's Pose 2 Seated Sun Salutation 3 Half Frog Pose 4 Locust Pose 5 Half Camel Pose 6 Child Pose	Self-love is the foundation of healing—but it can feel distant if you've been taught to prioritize others, dismiss your needs, or tie your worth to your performance. Without self-love, even small acts of care can feel undeserved.

Movement:

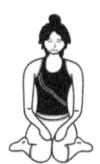

From your seat. Come to your **Hero's pose** on your shins. Put a block or pillow under your bottom for support, if that would feel better in your body.

Bring your hands together in front of your heart space, with your thumb knuckles connected to your sternum. Press into your thumb knuckles and feel this connection lift your heart forward.

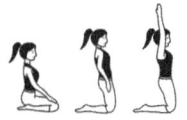

Pull your chin away from your chest. Inhale, lift your arms to the sky, shift your chin up, lift your gaze towards your hands. Exhale, palms come together—drag your hands back down to your heart. Pull your chin back down towards your chest to neutral. You may lift your body off of your knees or prop for more movement. Or stay lowered. Try both.

Repeat this **Seated Sun Salutation** 3 times.

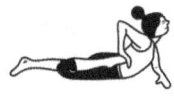

Slowly release your body down to your belly. Bend your left elbow, so your left forearm is parallel to the front of your mat. Hold it there. Bend your right knee as you reach your right arm around to the top of your right foot. Stay connected here and find a circular motion as you drag your foot out towards the right and eventually connect your right heel to your bottom. Press into your left forearm to find a small lift. **Half Frog pose**, right side.

Hold here for 5 breaths. Release your body down, find a reset with your breath. Prepare for the opposite side. Press your right forearm into the earth, bend your left knee, reach your left hand around to the top of your left foot. Slowly guide your left foot to your left in a circular motion, so your heel then reaches to your bottom. Press your right forearm into the earth to find lift. Half frog pose, left side. Hold here for 5 breaths.

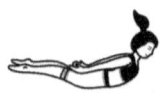

Release down onto your belly. Lengthen both arms, so they're by your sides and your palms are facing down. Press into the tops of your feet as you press the palms of your hands into the earth. Lift your chin away from your mat and find a small backbend, opening your heart and lifting you off the earth. Keep your gaze down and forward for 5 breaths. **Locust pose**. Repeat 3 times, with 5 intentional breaths in each round.

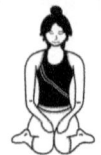

Come back into your **Hero's pose**, grab your blocks or two books and place them on both sides of your feet. Come to an upright position in your upper body leaving your shins on your mat with your toes flipped.

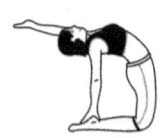

Reach your right hand towards your right heel or the book as you lift your left arm to the sky. Pull your torso up and to the sky as you drop your head back towards your shoulders. **Half Camel pose**, left side. Pause here for 3 breaths. Release back down into hero's pose, place your palms on your thighs, close your eyes and reset with 3 breaths.

Lift your heart, so it is above your hips, place your left hand to your left heel, with toes flipped. Reach your right arm to the sky and feel it reach behind you as you lift your chin up and open your throat. **Half camel pose**, right side. Hold here for 3 breaths.

Release your body back down into hero's pose. Face your palms up and reset with 5 breaths.

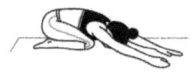
Slowly drop your heart toward the earth, keep your knees together and reach your arms around your shins, so your hands connect to your heels. **Child's pose.**

Hold here for five breaths.

Lift your body and come back into your easy seat.

Loving Yourself Like You Mean It – Self-Love Block / Barrier

Meditation (5 min):

Aham (I am)

Page 204

Repeat your mantra silently for 3–5 minutes, letting it anchor your awareness. If thoughts come, gently return to the mantra.

Remember: Thinking is only natural. Notice what arises—don't give it your attention.

Body-Based Reflections (5 min):

Use these prompts immediately after movement and meditation to stay connected to your body:

1. What happens in your body as you make space in your throat while in your half camel pose?

2. In the full expression of your camel pose, where do you feel the most sensation?

Reframe Limiting Thoughts (CBT) (5 min):

What came up for you today?

Refer back to pages: 213-218

- Limiting thought:

  _____

- Questions to ask:

  _____

- Reframed thought:

  _____

Healing Plans for the 14 Core Concerns

> **Be Curious...**
>
> Here are examples for your writing reflection, but feel free to pick your own.
>
> - Do I feel deserving of pleasure, rest, or being seen—just as I am?
> - How do these beliefs affect the way I receive touch, compliments, or desire?
> - Do I feel pressure to perform, please, or hide parts of myself?
> - How do these beliefs influence the kind of connection I seek—or avoid?

> **Affirmation to Anchor the Practice**
>
> *I deserve to love myself.*
>
> Repeat this affirmation silently or aloud as you close your practice. If it doesn't feel fully true yet—don't worry. Let it become a seed you're planting.

> *"When you give your thoughts space to stretch and your body space to feel, healing starts to speak."*

Healing What Wasn't Heard – Unrecognized Trauma

Breathwork (5 min):	Yoga Pose Flow (10 min):	What Unrecognized Trauma Looks Like
Ocean Breath Page 130	1 Seated Staff Pose 2 Reclined Figure 4 Pose 3 Mountain Pose 4 Forward Fold 5 Tree Pose	Old wounds that live in the body, even if your mind has tried to forget. You might feel triggered during intimacy, experience dissociation, or have unexplained tension or fear during certain movements or moments of closeness.

Movement:

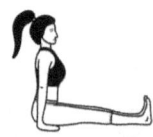

Find your seat with your legs straight in front of you. Feel both arms lengthen to the earth on each side of you to frame your body. Press your fingertips into the earth, so your arms straighten and your shoulders lift, so your heart can energetically shift forward. Flex your toes towards your face with effort as you engage your quads. Engage your core as you lengthen your spine. Hold here for 5 breaths in your **Seated Staff Pose**.

Repeat this 3 times, each with effort.

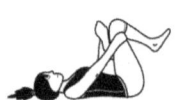

Lower onto your back and hug your knees into your chest. Plant your left foot on the earth, so your knee is reaching to the sky. Cross your right foot over your left knee and interlace your hands behind your left thigh. Stay here or lift your left foot, so your left knee is reaching towards your chest keeping the interlace behind your thigh. **Reclined Figure Four**, left side. Hold for 8 breaths.

Lower back down into your neutral pose. Rinse with your breath. Press your right foot into the earth, take your left foot and cross it over your right knee. Interlace your hands behind your right thigh. Stay here or pull your right knee towards your chest keeping the interlace behind your thigh. **Reclined Figure Four**, right side. Hold for 8 breaths.

Healing Plans for the 14 Core Concerns

Bring both knees into your chest and find a rock and roll motion up and down your spine until you're satisfied. Feel your way through it. Back and forth, rolling out any tension.

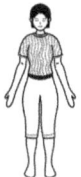

With this motion, use your momentum to lift up, and land in a standing **Mountain pose.** Inhale, lift your arms up to the sky. Exhale, release your arms down towards your hips, while simultaneously hinging at your hips to lower down into a **Forward Fold.**

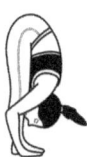

Create a sweeping motion here, a sun salutation movement of your own. You're moving from mountain pose, swinging your arms up, and lowering down into a forward fold. Find what feels good and repeat it 5 times.

When you're done, land in mountain pose. Reset. Breathe naturally for a few breaths.

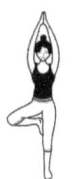

Pull your right knee into your chest and open your right hip, so your knee is reaching to your right. Connect your foot to the inside of your left thigh or the inside of your left calf or your left ankle for tree pose. Lift your arms to the sky, or bring your hands to your heart space. Hold for 8 breaths. **Tree pose**, right side.

Gently grab your knee, pull it back into your center line and hug your knee into your chest while you're standing, balancing on your left leg. Hold here for 2 breaths.

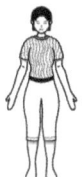

Release your right foot to the earth and come back to your mountain pose to find a release of your breath.

Ground down. Find your center. Stand tall.

Awaken Your Body Awaken Your Desire

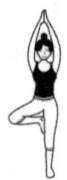

When you're ready, pull your left knee into your chest, open your left hip, so your left knee reaches to your left as you connect the inside of your left foot to the inside of your right thigh, calf or ankle. Place your hands to your heart or lift your arms to the sky. Feel your own expression of tree pose. Hold here balancing on your right leg for 8 breaths. **Tree pose**, left side.

Gently connect to your left knee and pull your left knee into your chest as you balance on your right foot. Hold here for 2 breaths.

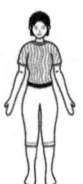

Release your left foot back down into your **Mountain pose**.

Close your eyes and reset with 3 breaths.

When ready, bring your body back into a comfortable seat.

Healing Plans for the 14 Core Concerns

Healing What Wasn't Heard – Unrecognized Trauma

Meditation (5 min):

Satya (Truth)
Page 203

Repeat your mantra silently for 3–5 minutes, letting it anchor your awareness. If thoughts come, gently return to the mantra.
Remember: Thinking is only natural. Notice what arises—don't give it your attention.

Body-Based Reflections (5 min):

Use these prompts immediately after movement and meditation to stay connected to your body:

1. Does folding forward or opening up feel better in your body?
2. What pose made you feel the most grounded?
3. What pose made you feel the safest in your body?

Reframe Limiting Thoughts (CBT) (5 min):

What came up for you today?

Refer back to pages: 213-218

- Limiting thought:

  _____

- Questions to ask:

  _____

- Reframed thought:

  _____

> **Be Curious...**

Here are examples for your writing reflection, but feel free to pick your own.

- Do I feel deserving of pleasure, rest, or being seen—just as I am?
- How do these beliefs affect the way I receive touch, compliments, or desire?
- Do I feel pressure to perform, please, or hide parts of myself?
- How do these beliefs influence the kind of connection I seek—or avoid?

> **Affirmation to Anchor the Practice**
>
> *I speak my truth without fear.*

Repeat this affirmation silently or aloud as you close your practice. If it doesn't feel fully true yet—don't worry. Let it become a seed you're planting.

"When you give your thoughts space to stretch and your body space to feel, healing starts to speak."

Chapter 17

Coming Home to Yourself

You made it.

Through pages of breath, movement, reflection, and rewiring—you stayed with yourself. You slowed down long enough to listen. You were brave enough to face what's been buried. You committed to create a new path forward.

That's no small thing.

Take a moment to reflect on what you've just done.

You've learned how to:

- Reconnect to your body through breath, movement, and stillness
- Anchor your awareness using mantra and sensation
- Identify the thoughts that no longer serve you—and replace them with ones that do
- Reclaim pleasure, safety, and desire—on your terms
- Create new beliefs about your worth, your sexuality, and your future

But more importantly, you've practiced what so many avoid: To be fully with yourself—without judgment.

This work is layered. It's not linear.

You may return to these practices again and again. And each time, you'll come back with more wisdom, more softness, and more clarity.

You don't need to be fully "healed" to live a meaningful, joyful life.

You don't need to fix everything before you can feel love or give love.

You are already worthy.

You are already whole.

A Few Final Encouragements

1. Progress is not about perfection.
   Some days your practice will feel like magic. Other days it might feel like a chore. Both count. Both are sacred.

2. Your pace is your power.
   Whether you move through one healing plan or five, you get to decide the rhythm. Trust your body's wisdom.

3. You're never behind.
   If you put the book down for a while, come back with fresh eyes. Nothing is lost. Your body remembers.

4. Celebrate the tiny wins.
   A shift in thought. A softening of breath. A moment of stillness. These are milestones.

Let It Keep Unfolding

Desire doesn't bloom on demand—it deepens with devotion. Not to someone else—but to yourself. The 30-day journey you're holding isn't a finish line—it's a foundation. A spark. A reintroduction to your body. When you reach the end of those thirty days, you may find that your healing is just getting started. Some seasons will ask you to linger longer. Others will invite bold expansion. Stay with it. Let

Coming Home to Yourself

your practice become a love affair—with your breath, your body, your becoming. This isn't the end. It's your awakening.

You've done something brave. You've done something beautiful.

As you close this chapter, know that the journey isn't ending—it's just beginning.

Keep listening.

Keep honoring.

Keep returning to yourself.

You're the safest place you'll ever know.

Trusted Clinical Resources

If you're seeking specialized support, these respected organizations offer directories of providers trained in sexual medicine, menopause care, and sex therapy. Each one can help you find informed, evidence-based care that aligns with your needs.

AASECT – *American Association of Sexuality Educators, Counselors and Therapists*

Find certified sex therapists, counselors, and educators trained in shame-free, research-based support for sexual wellness.

www.aasect.org

ISSWSH – *International Society for the Study of Women's Sexual Health*

A multidisciplinary network of clinicians and researchers specializing in women's sexual health, including desire, arousal, and pain conditions.

www.isswsh.org

NAMS – *North American Menopause Society*

Offers reliable, up-to-date resources on hormonal health and midlife care, plus a directory of certified menopause practitioners.

www.menopause.org

San Diego Sexual Medicine – *Led by Dr. Irwin Goldstein*

A leading clinical and research center dedicated to diagnosing and treating sexual pain and arousal concerns with an integrative approach.

www.sdsm.info

These resources are here to support you in finding care that's knowledgeable, respectful, and truly meets you where you are.

References

Babakhani, N., Taravati, M., Masoumi, Z., Garousian, M., Faradmal, J., & Shayan, A. (2018). The Effect of Cognitive-Behavioral Consultation on Sexual Function among Women: A Randomized Clinical Trial The Effect of Cognitive-Behavioral Consultation on Sexual Function among Women: A Randomized Clinical Trial. Journal of Caring Sciences, 7(2), 83–88. https://doi.org/10.15171/jcs.2018.013

Basson, R. (2000). *The female sexual response: A different model.* Journal of Sex & Marital Therapy, 26(1), 51–65. https://doi.org/10.1080/009262300278641

Berke, J. D. (2018). What does dopamine mean? Nature Neuroscience, 21(6), 787–793. https://doi.org/10.1038/s41593-018-0152-y

Boecker, H., Sprenger, T., Spilker, M. E., Henriksen, G., Koppenhoefer, M., Wagner, K. J., ... & Tolle, T. R. (2008). The runner's high: Opioidergic mechanisms in the human brain. Cerebral Cortex, 18(11), 2523–2531. https://doi.org/10.1093/cercor/bhn013

Brotto, L. A., Mehak, L., & Kit, C. (2009). Yoga and Sexual Functioning: A Review. Journal of Sex & Marital Therapy, 35(5), 378–390. https://doi.org/10.1080/00926230903065955

Chen, C. H., Lin, Y. C., Chiu, L. H., Chu, Y. H., Ruan, F. F., Liu, W. M., & Wang, P. H. (2013). Female sexual dysfunction: Definition, classification, and debates. Taiwanese Journal of Obstetrics and Gynecology, 52(1), 3–7. https://doi.org/10.1016/j.tjog.2013.01.002

Chudakov, B., Cohen, H., Matar, M. A., & Kaplan, Z. (2008). A Naturalistic Prospective Open Study of the Effects of Adjunctive Therapy of Sexual Dysfunction in Chronic PTSD Patients. A Naturalistic Prospective Open Study of the Effects of Adjunctive Therapy of Sexual Dysfunction in Chronic PTSD

Patients, 45(1), 26–32. Retrieved from https://doctorsonly.co.il/wp-content/uploads/2011/12/2008_1_5.pdf

Cleveland Clinic. (2021, December 10). Cortisol: What It Is, Function, Symptoms & Levels. Retrieved from https://my.clevelandclinic.org/health/articles/22187-cortisol

Cleveland Clinic. (2022, March 27). Epinephrine (Adrenaline): What It Is, Function, Deficiency & Side Effects. Retrieved from https://my.clevelandclinic.org/health/articles/22611-epinephrine-adrenaline

Dhikav, V., Karmarkar, G., Gupta, R., Verma, M., Gupta, R., Gupta, S., & Anand, K. S. (2010). Yoga in Female Sexual Functions. The Journal of Sexual Medicine, 7(2), 964–970. https://doi.org/10.1111/j.1743-6109.2009.01580.x

Dishman, R. K., & O'Connor, P. J. (2009). Lessons in exercise neurobiology: The case of endorphins. Mental Health and Physical Activity, 2(1), 4–9. https://doi.org/10.1016/j.mhpa.2009.01.002

Dossett, M. L., Fricchione, G. L., & Benson, H. (2020). A New Era for Mind–Body Medicine. New England Journal of Medicine, 382(15), 1390–1391. https://doi.org/10.1056/nejmp1917461

Durna, G., Ülbe, S., & Dirik, G. (2020). Mindfulness-Based Interventions in the Treatment of Female Sexual Dysfunction: A Systemic Review. Psikiyatride Guncel Yaklasimlar - Current Approaches in Psychiatry, 12(1), 72–90. https://doi.org/10.18863/pgy.470683

Dusek, J. A., & Benson, H. (2009). Mind-body medicine: a model of the comparative clinical impact of the acute stress and relaxation responses. Minnesota medicine, 92(5), 47–50. Retrieved from www.ncbi.nlm.nih.gov/MusePath/pmc/articles/PMC2724877/

Fisher, H. E., Xu, X., Aron, A., & Brown, L. L. (2016). Intense, Passionate, Romantic Love: A Natural Addiction? How the Fields That Investigate Romance and Substance Abuse Can Inform Each Other. Frontiers in Psychology, 7. https://doi.org/10.3389/fpsyg.2016.00687

Frühauf, S., Gerger, H., Schmidt, H. M., Munder, T., & Barth, J. (2013). Efficacy of Psychological Interventions for Sexual Dysfunction: A Systematic Review and Meta-Analysis. Archives of Sexual Behavior, 42(6), 915–933. https://doi.org/10.1007/s10508-012-0062-0

References

Goldstein, I., Pfaus, J. G., & Kim, N. N. (2006). Toward a better understanding of the biology of female sexual function. In I. Goldstein, C. M. Meston, S. R. Davis, & A. Traish (Eds.), *Textbook of female sexual dysfunction* (pp. 69–84). Taylor & Francis.

Gordon, B., Chen, M. Y., Durstine, J. L., & Mahalakshmi, B. (2017). Exercise and hormonal regulation. Endocrine Connections, 6(8), R208–R227. https://doi.org/10.1530/EC-17-0103

Gotink, R. A., Vernooij, M. W., Ikram, M. A., Niessen, W. J., Krestin, G. P., Hofman, A., Hunink, M. G. M. (2018). Meditation and yoga practice are associated with smaller right amygdala volume: the Rotterdam study. Brain Imaging and Behavior, 12(6), 1631–1639. https://doi.org/10.1007/s11682-018-9826-z

Hackney, A. C. (2020). Exercise as a stressor to the human neuroendocrine system. Hormones, 19(4), 419–431. https://doi.org/10.1007/s42000-020-00209-7

Hamilton, L. D., & Meston, C. M. (2013). Chronic Stress and Sexual Function in Women. The Journal of Sexual Medicine, 10(10), 2443–2454. https://doi.org/10.1111/jsm.12249

Hamilton, L. D., Rellini, A. H., & Meston, C. M. (2008). Cortisol, Sexual Arousal, and Affect in Response to Sexual Stimuli. The Journal of Sexual Medicine, 5(9), 2111–2118. https://doi.org/10.1111/j.1743-6109.2008.00922.x

Harris, G. (1970). Effects of the Nervous System on Pituitary—Adrenal Activity. Progress in Brain Research, 86–88. https://doi.org/10.1016/s0079-6123(08)61522-8

Haynes, T. (2018, May 1). Dopamine, Smartphones & You: A battle for your time. Retrieved from https://sitn.hms.harvard.edu/flash/2018/dopamine-smartphones-battle-time/

Hiller-Strumhöfel, S., & Bartke, A. (1998). The Endocrine System: An Overview. Alcohol Health & Research World, 22(3), 153–164. Retrieved from https://www.ncbi.nlm.nih.gov/MusePath/pmc/articles/PMC6761896/pdf/arh-22-3-153.pdf

Joseph, D., & Whirledge, S. (2017). Stress and the HPA Axis: Balancing Homeostasis and Fertility. International Journal of Molecular Sciences, 18(10), 2224. https://doi.org/10.3390/ijms18102224

Kabat-Zinn, J. (2005). Coming to Our Senses. Amsterdam, Netherlands: Adfo Books.

Kaushik, M., Jain, A., Agarwal, P., Joshi, S. D., & Parvez, S. (2020). Role of Yoga and Meditation as Complimentary Therapeutic Regime for Stress-Related Neuropsychiatric Disorders: Utilization of Brain Waves Activity as Novel Tool. Journal of Evidence-Based Integrative Medicine, 25, 2515690X2094945. https://doi.org/10.1177/2515690x20949451

Khalsa, M. K., Greiner-Ferris, J. M., Hofmann, S. G., & Khalsa, S. B. S. (2014). Yoga-Enhanced Cognitive Behavioural Therapy (Y-CBT) for Anxiety Management: A Pilot Study. Clinical Psychology & Psychotherapy, 22(4), 364–371. https://doi.org/10.1002/cpp.1902

Komisaruk, B. R., Beyer-Flores, C., & Whipple, B. (2006). The science of orgasm. Baltimore, MD: Johns Hopkins University Press.

Krieger, J. F., Kristensen, E., Marquardsen, M., & Giraldi, A. (2019). Mindfulness in the treatment of sexual dysfunction. Retrieved from https://ugeskriftet.dk/videnskab/mindfulness-i-behandlingen-af-seksuelle-funktionsforstyrrelser

Krishnakumar, D., Hamblin, M. R., & Lakshmanan, S. (2015). Meditation and Yoga can Modulate Brain Mechanisms that affect Behavior and Anxiety- A Modern Scientific Perspective. Ancient Science, 2(1), 13–19. https://doi.org/10.14259/as.v2i1.171

Laine, C. M., Valtonen, E. J., Helminen, E. E., & Laaksonen, D. E. (2016). The effect of physical activity on vascular endothelial function. Physiology & Behavior, 164(Pt B), 362–368. https://doi.org/10.1016/j.physbeh.2016.05.038

Lehmiller, J. J., Garcia, J. R., Gesselman, A. N., & Mark, K. P. (2020). Less Sex, but More Sexual Diversity: Changes in Sexual Behavior during the COVID-19 Coronavirus Pandemic. Leisure Sciences, 43(1–2), 295–304. https://doi.org/10.1080/01490400.2020.1774016

Leonti, M., & Casu, L. (2018). Ethnopharmacology of Love. Frontiers in Pharmacology, 9. https://doi.org/10.3389/fphar.2018.00567

Masoudi, M., Maasoumi, R., & Bragazzi, N. L. (2022). Effects of the COVID-19 pandemic on sexual functioning and activity: a systematic review and meta-analysis. BMC Public Health, 22(1). https://doi.org/10.1186/s12889-021-12390-4

McEwen, B. S. (2017). Neurobiological and Systemic Effects of Chronic Stress. Chronic Stress, 1, 247054701769232. https://doi.org/10.1177/2470547017692328

References

McEwen, B. S., Gray, J. D., & Nasca, C. (2015). 60 Years Of Neuroendocrinology: Redefining neuroendocrinology: stress, sex and cognitive and emotional regulation. Journal of Endocrinology, 226(2), T67–T83. https://doi.org/10.1530/joe-15-0121

Porges, S. W. (2007). The polyvagal perspective. Biological Psychology, 74(2), 116–143. https://doi.org/10.1016/j.biopsycho.2006.06.009

Rosen, R. C., Connor, M. K., Miyasato, G., Link, C., Shifren, J. L., Fisher, W. A., Schobelock, M. J. (2012). Sexual Desire Problems in Women Seeking Healthcare: A Novel Study Design for Ascertaining Prevalence of Hypoactive Sexual Desire Disorder in Clinic-Based Samples of U.S. Women. Journal of Women's Health, 21(5), 505–515. https://doi.org/10.1089/jwh.2011.3002

Rizvi, S. J., & Kennedy, S. H. (2013). Management strategies for SSRI-induced sexual dysfunction. Journal of psychiatry & neuroscience: JPN, 38(5), E27–E28. https://doi.org/10.1503/jpn.130076

Salmon, P. (2001). Effects of physical exercise on anxiety, depression, and sensitivity to stress: A unifying theory. Clinical Psychology Review, 21(1), 33–61. https://doi.org/10.1016/S0272-7358(99)00032-X

Seshadri, K. (2016). The neuroendocrinology of love. Indian Journal of Endocrinology and Metabolism, 20(4), 558. https://doi.org/10.4103/2230-8210.183479

Simon, N. M., Hofmann, S. G., Rosenfield, D., Hoeppner, S. S., Hoge, E. A., Bui, E., & Khalsa, S. B. S. (2021). Efficacy of Yoga vs Cognitive Behavioral Therapy vs Stress Education for the Treatment of Generalized Anxiety Disorder. JAMA Psychiatry, 78(1), 13. https://doi.org/10.1001/jamapsychiatry.2020.2496

Smith, S. M., & Vale, W. W. (2006). The role of the hypothalamic-pituitary-adrenal axis in neuroendocrine responses to stress. Dialogues in Clinical Neuroscience, 8(4), 383–395. https://doi.org/10.31887/dcns.2006.8.4/ssmith

Streeter, C. C., Gerbarg, P. L., Saper, R. B., Ciraulo, D. A., & Brown, R. P. (2012). Effects of yoga on the autonomic nervous system, gamma-aminobutyric-acid, and allostasis in epilepsy, depression, and post-traumatic stress disorder. Journal of Alternative and Complementary Medicine, 18(8), 800– 807. https://doi.org/10.1089/acm.2011.0268

Swanson, A. (2019). Science of Yoga: Understand the Anatomy and Physiology to Perfect Your Practice (Annotated ed.). New York, NY: DK Publishing.

Tindle, J., & Tadi, P. (2021). Neuroanatomy, Parasympathetic Nervous System. In StatPearls. StatPearls Publishing. https://www.ncbi.nlm.nih.gov/books/NBK553141/

Trainor, B. C. (2011). Stress responses and the mesolimbic dopamine system: Social contexts and sex differences. Hormones and Behavior, 60(5), 457–469. https://doi.org/10.1016/j.yhbeh.2011.08.013

Tsatsoulis, A., & Fountoulakis, S. (2006). The protective role of exercise on stress system dysregulation and comorbidities. Annals of the New York Academy of Sciences, 1083(1), 196–213. https://doi.org/10.1196/annals.1367.020

van Anders, S. M., Herbenick, D., Brotto, L. A., Harris, E. A., & Chadwick, S. B. (2021). The Heteronormativity Theory of Low Sexual Desire in Women Partnered with Men. Archives of Sexual Behavior, 51(1), 391–415. https://doi.org/10.1007/s10508-021-02100-x

Wallace, R., Benson, H., & Wilson, A. (1971). A wakeful hypometabolic physiologic state. American Journal of Physiology-Legacy Content, 221(3), 795–799. https://doi.org/10.1152/ajplegacy.1971.221.3.795

Williams, O. O. F., Coppolino, M., George, S. R., & Perreault, M. L. (2021). Sex Differences in Dopamine Receptors and Relevance to Neuropsychiatric Disorders. Brain Sciences, 11(9), 1199. https://doi.org/10.3390/brainsci11091199

www.ingramcontent.com/pod-product-compliance
Lightning Source LLC
Chambersburg PA
CBHW020454030426
42337CB00011B/105